SIMPLE & SAFE BABY-LED WEANING

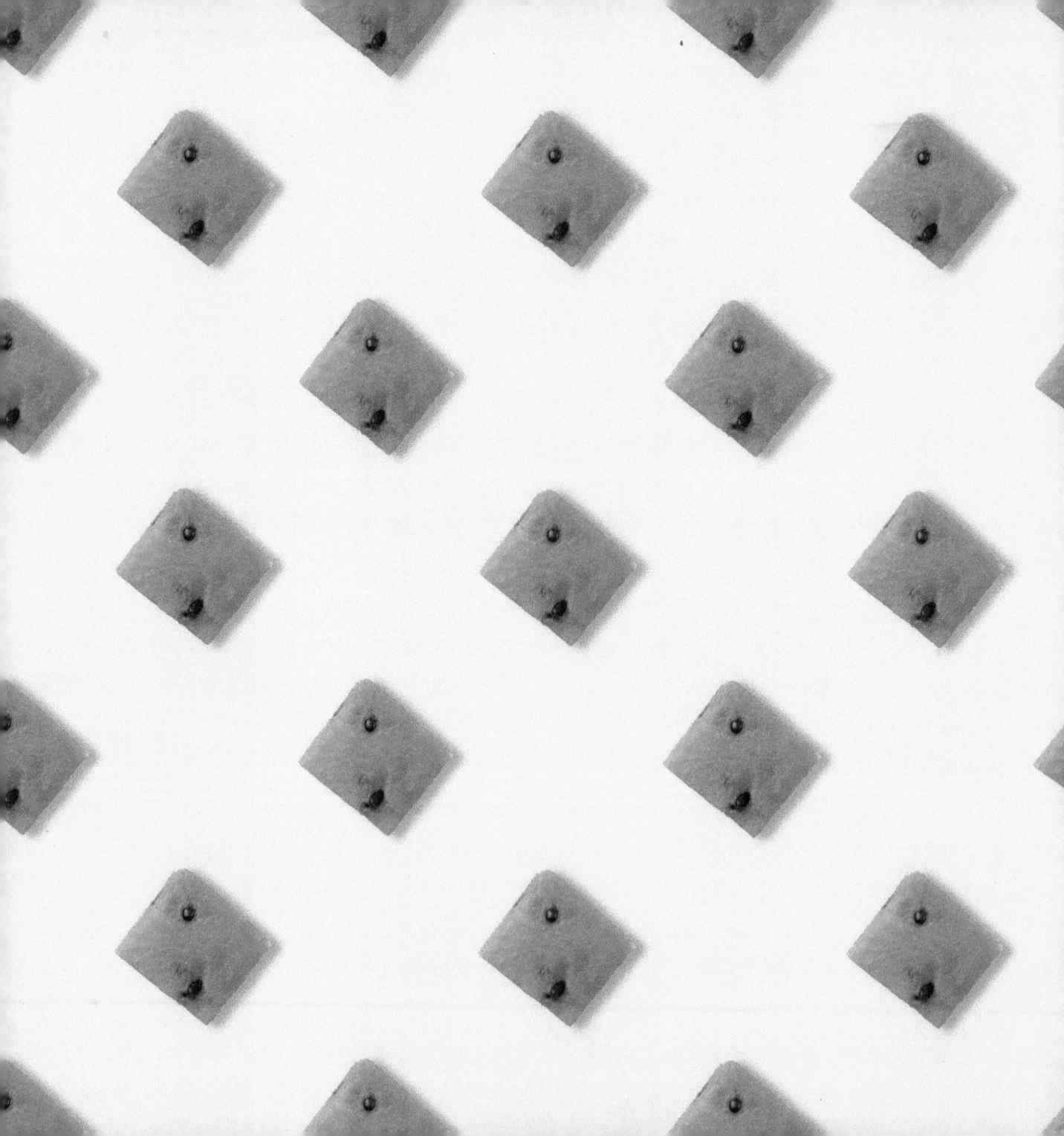

SIMPLE & SAFE
BABY-LED WEANING

How to Integrate Foods, Master Portion Sizes, and Identify Allergies

MALINA LINKAS MALKANI, MS, RDN, CDN

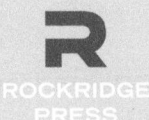

ROCKRIDGE
PRESS

To my girls, Alienna, Evangeline, and Solenne,
who will always be my babies.

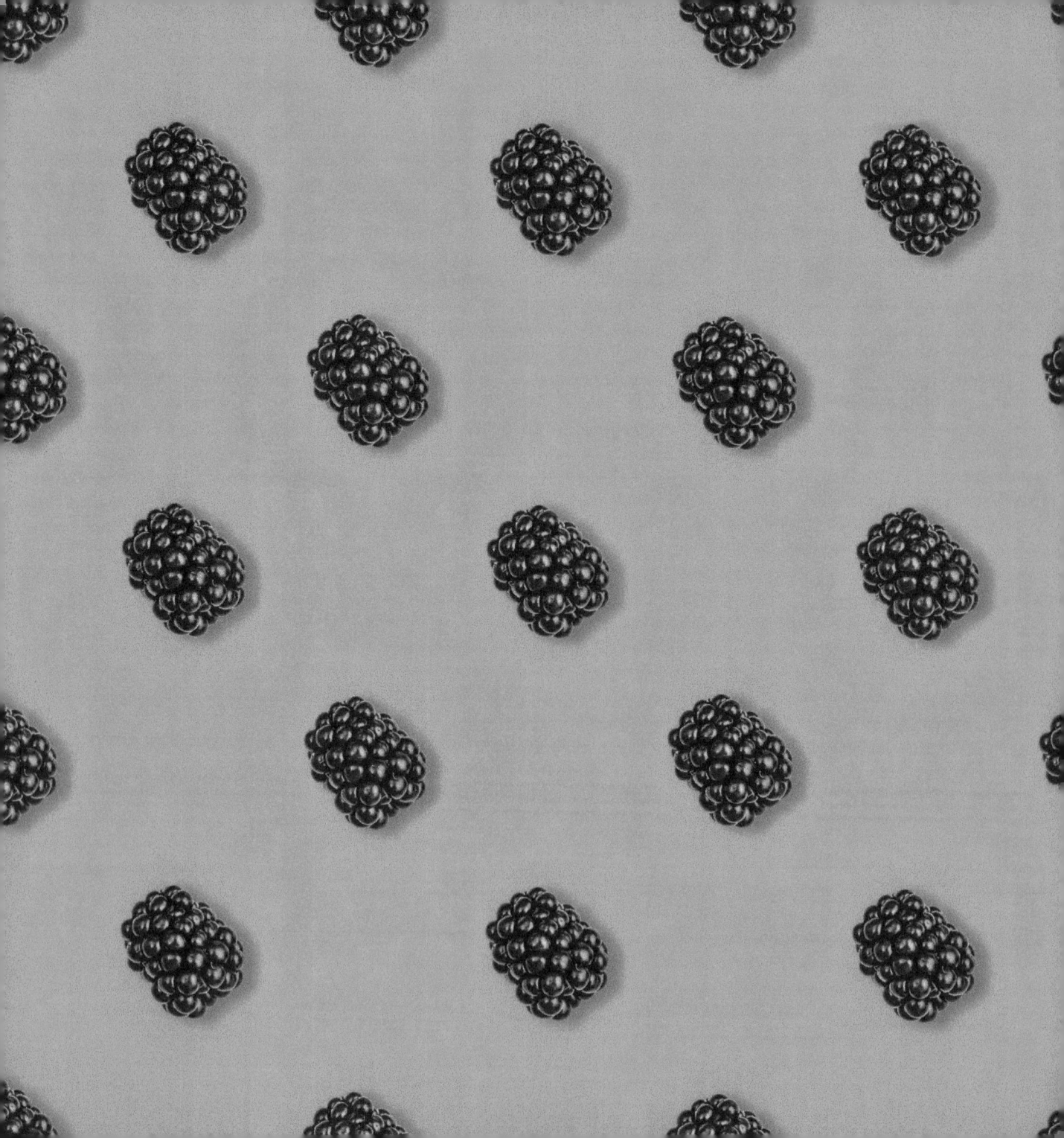

CONTENTS

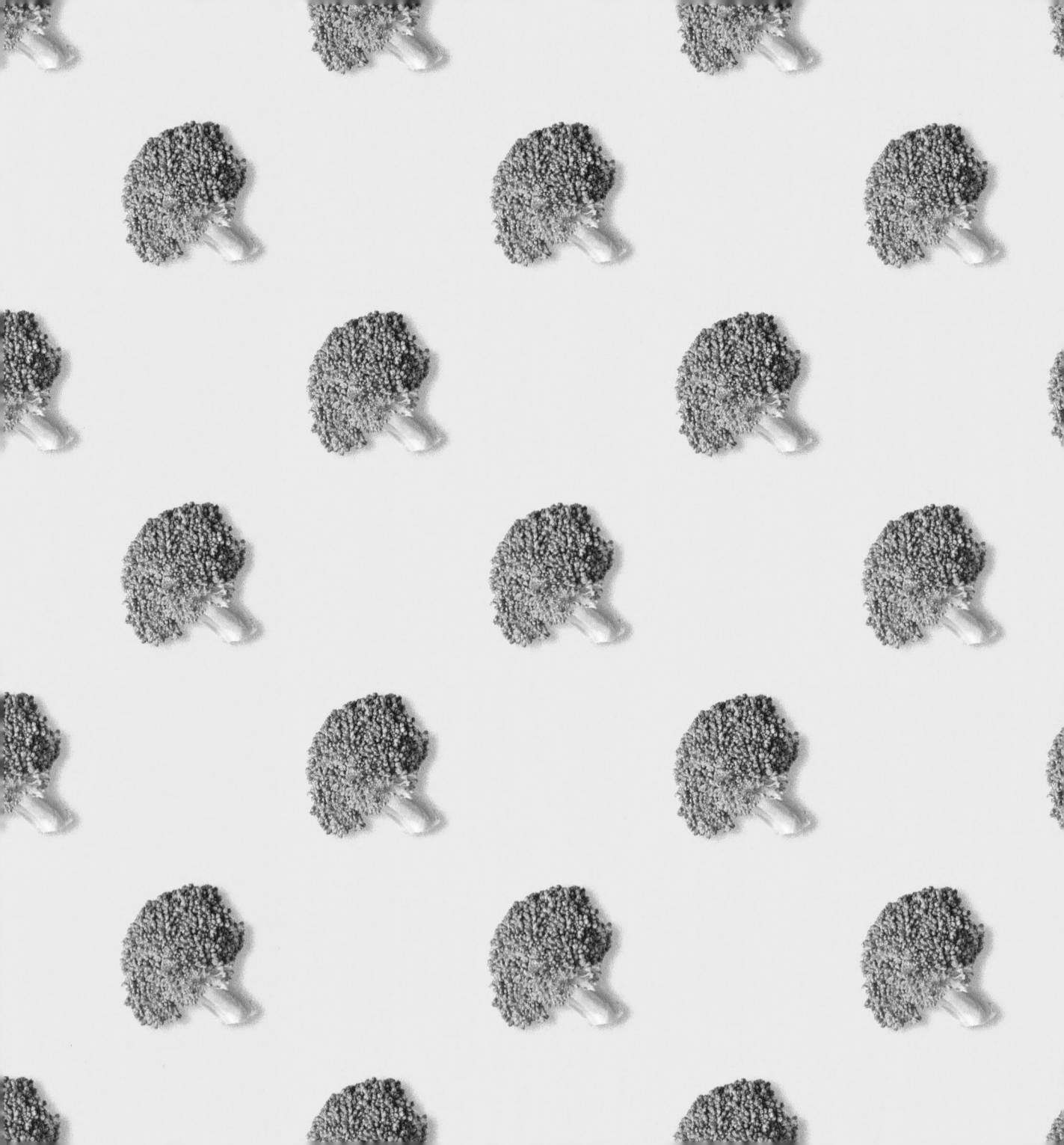

INTRODUCTION

If you are reading this book, it is likely that it is almost time to introduce your baby to one of the most enjoyable pleasures in life—eating real solid food! Kudos to you for considering baby-led weaning (BLW) as an approach to feeding. You may have read or heard that BLW babies are less likely to become picky eaters, or that BLW is a simpler, more affordable path than navigating jarred baby food and ice-cube trays of frozen purées. You may also have some apprehension regarding the safety and practicality of BLW—which, by the way, is very normal. With this book, it is my goal to help answer all of your questions and concerns so that when the time is right, you feel prepared and confident to start your little one on solid foods using BLW.

My experience with BLW is both personal and professional. I am a licensed, registered dietitian nutritionist and the founder of Malina Malkani, LLC. I am also a mom of three young children who were all born within a few years of one another, so I have spent a lot of time feeding babies and of course preparing meals—all while juggling an infant in a sling, perching a toddler on my hip, and dodging the third one racing around the kitchen! In both my home and work life, I have seen that BLW supports a baby's ability to self-nourish, self-feed, and self-regulate food intake, all of which helps establish the foundation for a lifelong healthy relationship with food.

In my private practice and nutrition consulting company, I focus on helping parents provide more nutrient-dense, minimally processed whole foods for their kids—a lifestyle I created and trademarked called "Wholitarian" (pronounced "WHOLE-tarian"). I originally developed the term and concept for my clients as a way to quickly and easily reference a dietary pattern focused on minimally processed plant-based foods (vegetables, fruits, whole grains, nuts, seeds, beans, and legumes). Experts agree that not only are these foods best for longevity and protection against many chronic diseases, but they also provide high-quality nutrition and a variety of textures for your baby as you begin your journey with BLW.

Although a Wholitarian lifestyle is built around plant-based foods, it does not necessarily have to be vegan or even vegetarian. It is flexible and does not prohibit the inclusion of some dairy foods and nondairy alternatives, occasional meat and poultry dishes, and even hamburgers and birthday cake every once in a while. It allows for the realities and stresses of family life, recognizing that when you eat healthy, balanced meals most of the time, it is fine to occasionally feed the family boxed mac and cheese when time is tight. Generally speaking, this approach to food and nutrition complements BLW by establishing a balanced approach to healthy eating at mealtimes—meals in which your baby will soon participate.

One of the most attractive aspects of BLW is that your baby can eat what you eat—with a few simple modifications—and thus be included in family meals. This makes the entire process of meal preparation and planning easier, less expensive, and less time-consuming. The best-kept secret of all is that making one meal for everyone is not only more convenient for parents, but also healthier for your baby (and your other children, too).

In my nutrition practice, I see many parents who are stressed about how and what to feed their kids. They struggle with picky eaters, eating habits that have gotten off-track, and concerns about nutrient deficiencies. BLW helps reduce parents' anxiety about feeding their babies, because unlike a conventional approach, the "what" and "how" of BLW form the foundation of long-term healthy eating habits. With the practice of family meals firmly in place from the beginning, babies generally grow into more adventurous, healthy eaters, and families can avoid many common nutrition-related issues down the road.

With this book, my goal is to provide simple, straightforward guidance on how to safely integrate BLW into your family life so you can enjoy this wonderful stage in your baby's development and reap all the long-term benefits of BLW without worry. To this end, I include information on how to determine whether your baby is ready to start solids and what to expect once you do begin. At the heart of the book is all the practical advice you will need to get started with BLW, including how to safely prepare and store your baby's food, a list of 26 ideal foods to start with, and how to combine them into balanced meals. I also cover what foods to avoid, how to recognize the difference between gagging and choking, and what to do about both. All along the way, I include nutrition information, helpful tips, and a variety of photos that help clarify the process.

Introducing solid foods to your baby's diet can come with some level of concern about food allergies, so I include a detailed discussion about food allergies and sensitivities and how to navigate them during BLW. You will find information on the eight major allergens, what to look for in terms of allergic reactions, and what to do if you think your baby may be allergic to something. After reading this book, you will have all the tools and information you need to successfully tackle this exciting new stage in your baby's life. Let's get started!

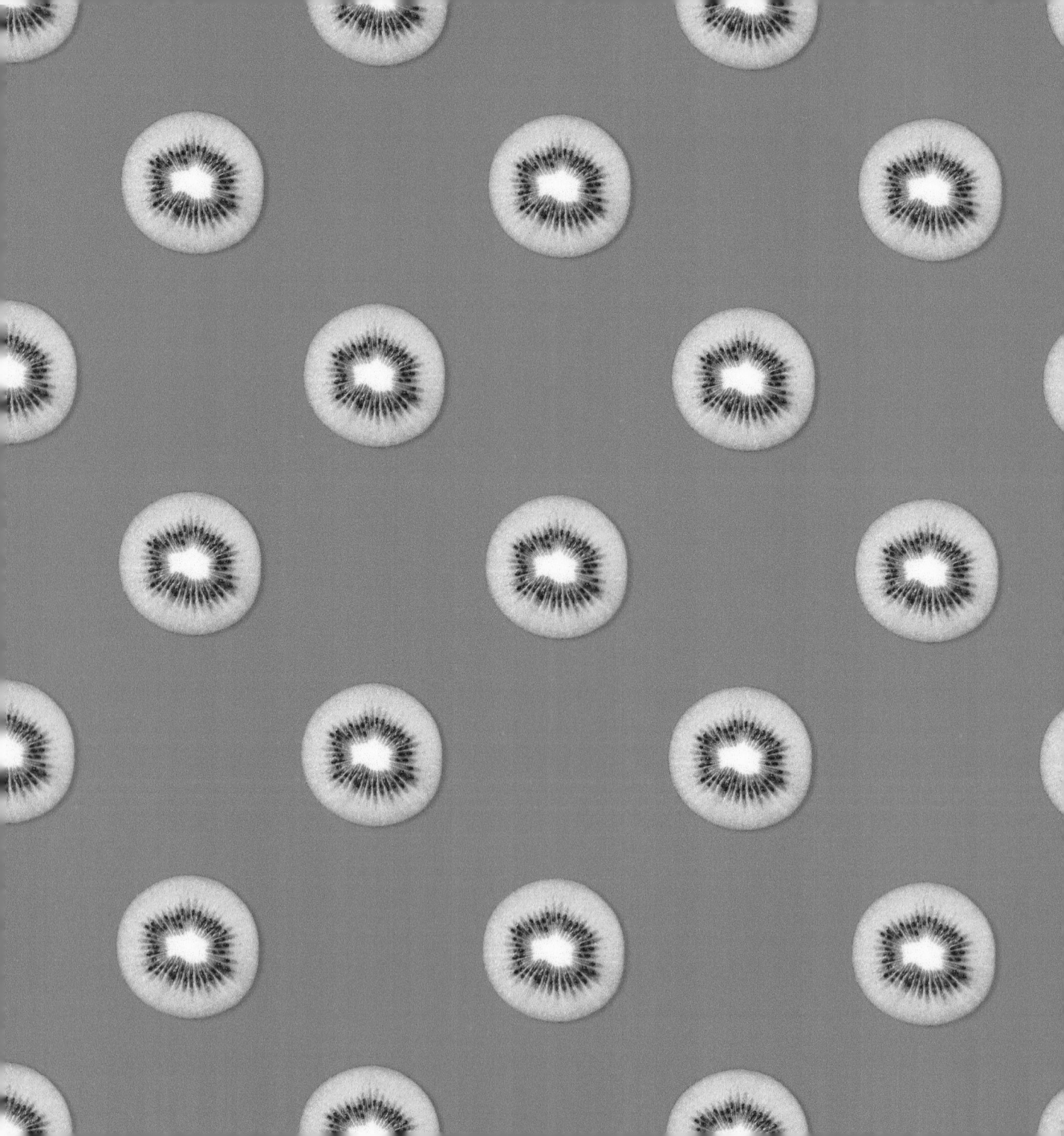

PART ONE

BABY-LED WEANING 101

If you are feeling overwhelmed, please know that you are not alone. Although this phase in your baby's development can be gratifying (and at times hilarious), it can also feel nerve-racking, especially in the beginning. Even as a food and nutrition expert with a graduate degree in clinical nutrition, I agonized over when to start solids with my first child. Feeling overwhelmed is a common and natural reaction to this change in the way you will nourish and care for your baby. But take heart—soon you will have all the guidance you need to feed your baby safely, completely, and conveniently.

You might be a little curious about the difference between the terms "baby-led weaning" and "baby-led feeding," which are sometimes used interchangeably. Baby-led weaning refers to the method of infant feeding that skips the spoon-feeding of purées and instead involves offering babies appropriately sized finger foods for self-feeding at the family table starting at about 6 months of age.

However, the "weaning" aspect of the term "baby-led weaning" can be somewhat confusing, since many people associate weaning with the transition away from breast milk or formula, when in fact baby-led weaning involves a baby continuing to drink formula or breast milk (in addition to eating finger foods) until at least 12 months of age.

The most fundamental aspect of baby-led weaning is not actually "weaning" but "baby-led," which is why many experts prefer to call the feeding method "baby-led feeding." Whatever you choose to call it, the most important part is that your baby is self-feeding, has control over food intake, and actively self-regulates rather than being passively spoon-fed by an adult.

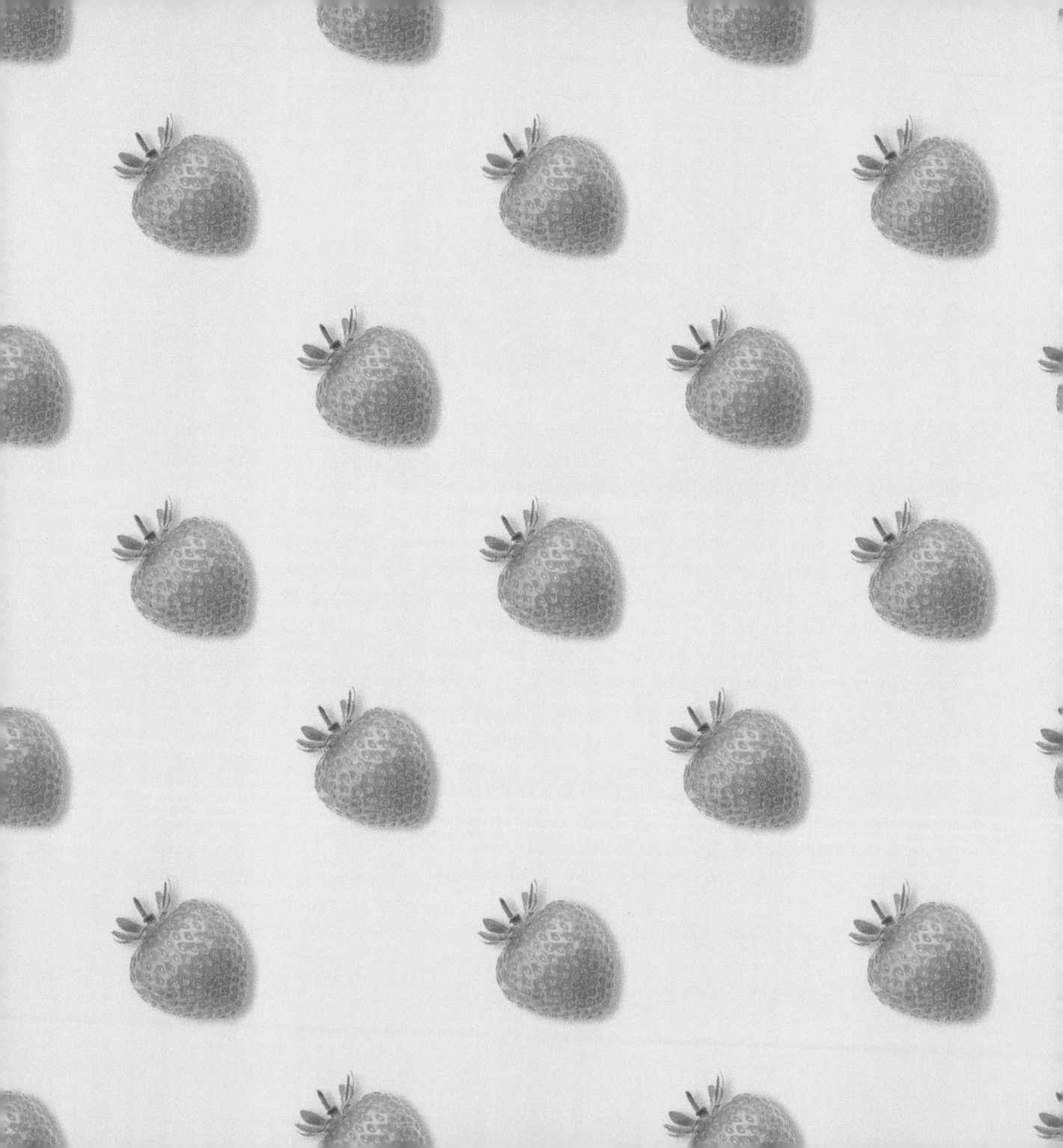

CHAPTER ONE

BABY-LED WEANING IS NOTHING NEW

It may help to know that BLW is not a new approach. It has been steadily gaining in popularity ever since the groundbreaking publication of the book *Baby-Led Weaning* by Gill Rapley and Tracey Murkett in 2008. Parents from around the world and throughout history have offered babies finger foods from the family table. According to research conducted by Rachel Howcroft at Stockholm University in 2013, for example, hunter-gatherers once offered their babies mashed fish and meat with animal fat. A chapter from the book *Weaning: Why, What, and When?* reports that babies in various regions of Africa are typically offered foods that are left over from the meals prepared for adults. And, according to research conducted in 2011 by Julie Tate of East Tennessee State University, infants in Mongolia are given smaller, bite-size portions of whatever foods the rest of the family is eating. A 2014 study in the *Pan American Journal of Public Health* reports that the inaugural foods of babies growing up in the Peruvian Amazon include potatoes, bananas, grains, and porridge.

In Western cultures, however, spoon-feeding purées has been the norm for many decades, perhaps for the wrong reasons. Guidance on when to start feeding solids to babies has changed many times throughout the 20th century, reflecting misguided advice from health professionals and shifting recommendations on breastfeeding and formula feeding. In the early 1900s, doctors instructed mothers to breastfeed on a strict schedule with a number of hours between nursings, as they did not yet understand that frequent breastfeeding was necessary to stimulate milk production. As a result, many mothers could not make enough milk to satisfy their hungry babies, and consequently infant "solids" (mostly cereals) were recommended for babies as young as 2 months old. These solids had to be spoon-fed because the babies receiving them were so young that they could not yet feed themselves, which led to a cultural assumption that spoon-feeding is the only way to start babies on solid foods. Perhaps as a culture, this excessively early introduction of solids that necessitated spoon-feeding is a part of how we got off-track in self-regulating our food intake and acknowledging our internal cues for hunger and fullness.

By the 1950s, as more women joined the workforce, the commercialized baby food industry began marketing jarred purées as a superior source of nourishment and a convenient product for modern moms. In the 1960s, it was normal to start babies on purées at 2 to 3 months of age, whereas in the 1990s it became closer to 4 months. It was not until the World Health Organization (WHO) changed its recommendation in 2002 to offering solids starting from 6 months, while applying responsive feeding techniques (the practice of recognizing a baby's cues for hunger and fullness and responding appropriately to those cues) that the BLW movement began to take off.

The funny thing is that, recommendations aside, many parents with multiple kids stumble onto BLW out of necessity. This was my experience. With my first daughter, I followed all the "rules" and started her on purées when she was 4 months old. She progressed through the different stages and onto finger foods, and she was frankly a rather picky eater as a toddler.

Less than two years later, when my second child came along, I was more seasoned and less afraid to offer her finger foods from the family meal, especially since she seemed to relish feeding herself and was generally irritated whenever anyone tried to spoon-feed her. By the time my third child was born a little more than a year later, like many other parents, I was too busy caring for my young children to listen to recommendations that went against what experience had taught me.

By then, I trusted that babies are—from the title of Leslie Schilling and Wendy Jo Peterson's wonderful book—*Born to Eat*, and that their self-feeding and fine motor skills emerge and develop when they are ready to start solids. When my youngest was 6 months old, I mostly skipped purées and offered modified versions of whatever we were eating, marveling at the power of family meals and role modeling as I watched her mimic her older sisters eating finger foods at the family table. Can you guess which one of my daughters was my fussiest eater throughout early childhood? If you guessed my oldest, you are right.

Picky Little Eaters

One of the most common nutrition-related struggles I see among parents is how to deal with picky eating in children. For many parents it comes as a shock when their child, who was a champion eater as an infant, hits toddlerhood and suddenly refuses certain foods.

This change is normal. Picky eating tends to come and go throughout the toddler and preschool years, peaking at about 20 months of age and most often resolving by about age 6. From a developmental perspective, picky eating usually emerges as an expression of a toddler's desire to exert independence. During a time of life when much is decided for them, toddlers soon discover that food is a way to take control, express opinions, investigate cause and effect, and communicate dissatisfaction. By about age 6, most kids have developed more effective ways to communicate and express their individuality, and picky eating habits start to fade.

Despite best intentions, the way parents and caregivers react to picky eating tends to affect whether it decreases, intensifies, or sticks around even longer. The good news is that BLW helps establish positive feeding practices early on, and it consequently minimizes picky eating in later years. These practices include the following:

- Participating in as many family meals as possible
- Establishing a strong division of responsibility in which parents decide the **what**, **when**, and **where** of meals and kids decide **whether** and **how much** to eat
- Implementing a solid but flexible schedule of three meals a day with a couple of snacks in between and no grazing
- Not giving up if a child refuses a new food—not pressing it in the moment, but instead offering the food again repeatedly, at different meals and prepared in a variety of ways
- Never pressuring, cajoling, bribing, or forcing kids to eat

If, as your baby grows into toddlerhood, you find yourself concerned that you may have a picky eater on your hands, double down on the foundational principles of BLW—which are powerful in babyhood and beyond.

Why Start Baby-Led Weaning?

You may already be familiar with some of the nutrition-related benefits of BLW, but there are additional advantages that involve other aspects of health. Sure, starting solids using a BLW approach increases the likelihood that your baby will eat a greater number of minimally processed, nutrient-dense, fresh foods that help support growth and development. But what sets BLW apart from a conventional approach is the impact of responsive feeding on self-regulation. (Remember that responsive feeding is the practice of recognizing a baby's cues for hunger and fullness and responding appropriately to those cues.)

According to a 2016 study published in the journal *BMJ Open*, self-feeding in BLW strengthens a baby's ability to self-regulate food intake and helps them integrate earlier into family meals. A 2012 study in the same publication found that BLW promotes healthy food preferences and less picky eating in early childhood. Research findings from 2017 in both *JAMA Pediatrics* and *PLOS ONE* also suggest that BLW leads to more adventurous eating and less food fussiness.

BLW boosts babies' fine motor skills and dexterity and stimulates babies with new shapes, colors, textures, and flavors. It also saves money and time since, with some minor adjustments, the whole family eats the same food at meals, setting the stage for the entire family to enjoy a lifelong, healthier relationship with food.

How Do I Know When It Is Time for My Baby to Start Baby-Led Weaning?

Guidelines on when to start solid foods have changed a lot over the past 50 years or so, and even now there are some conflicting recommendations, all of which make the question of when to start solids confusing for parents. Recent studies in the *Italian Journal of Pediatrics* and the *American Journal of Preventive Medicine* suggest that introducing solids too early may increase obesity risk. On the other hand, starting solids too late might lead to delayed oral motor function and food or texture aversions. It also increases the risk for food allergies, nutrient deficiencies, and poorer diets down the road.

For example, the iron reserves of full-term babies are typically exhausted at the age of 6 months; after that, babies need iron-containing foods to meet their iron needs. Without them, babies this age and older are at risk for iron-deficiency anemia, which can affect overall health, reduce immune system function, and cause irreversible delays in cognitive development.

In response to the newest research, the majority of health organizations agree that starting a baby on solid foods before 4 months is too early and that after 7 months is too late. The WHO, the American Academy of Pediatrics, and the Academy of Nutrition and Dietetics all recommend introducing complementary foods to babies from or around 6 months of age. Waiting until about 6 months to start solids means that spoon-feeding is not necessary, given the difference in self-feeding skills between a child who is 3 to 4 months old and one who is 6 months old.

This does not mean that you should automatically offer solids on your baby's 6-month birthday. Look for signs that indicate a readiness for solid foods. If you do not observe them and your baby is at least 6 months old, wait another week and reassess. If your baby was born prematurely, it may take until she reaches the age of 6 months from what would have been the full-term due date for these signs to develop.

Signs That Indicate Readiness for Solid Foods

The following specific signs of readiness indicate that your baby can try starting solid foods:

- Maintains an upright sitting position with minimal support
- Holds the head and neck still while seated
- Takes an interest in food and eating
- Grabs larger objects and brings them to the mouth
- Tongue thrust reflex has disappeared

Be sure to communicate closely with your pediatrician throughout the process of starting solids. Luckily, there are about seven recommended pediatrician visits throughout a baby's first year of life, which offer multiple opportunities to ask about and discuss your child's development and readiness for solid foods.

Signs That Do NOT Indicate Readiness for Solid Foods

The following behaviors and traits are developmentally normal but do not indicate readiness for solid foods:

- Makes lip-smacking sounds
- No longer falls asleep right after drinking breastmilk or formula
- Wakes throughout the night
- Seems comparatively small (or big)
- Weight gain has slowed
- Has some teeth

For some babies, BLW may not be the best fit. This includes preterm babies and babies with medical or developmental delays who may tolerate puréed textures better, or need further oral or sensory assessments and are best assessed on a case-by-case basis. Babies who are at high risk for food allergies may need to preventively start solids as early as 4 months, in which case finger foods are not advised.

If, for whatever reason, you find that BLW is not for you and your baby, that is okay! Know that using a conventional feeding method is a viable and valid option as well. A spoon-fed baby (and especially one who is fed responsively) can be just as well-nourished and adventurous as a BLW-fed baby, and many parents prefer a combined approach involving both purées and finger foods. In any case, BLW is simply an approach to infant feeding that many parents find works better for them and has the advantage of providing a foundation for healthy eating habits down the road.

Developmental Milestones: Palmar and Pincer Grasps

Palmar and pincer grasps are milestones in a baby's fine motor development. The palmar grasp typically develops first, followed by the pincer grasp. The type of grasp your baby uses influences the size and shape of finger foods you offer.

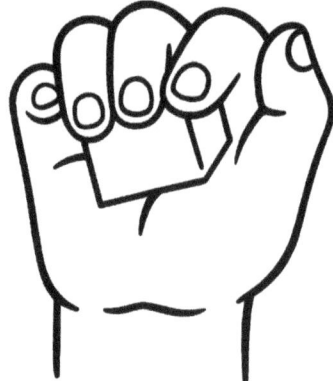

Palmar grasp: *"Palming" an object or curling the fingers around an object and in toward the palm of the hand.*

Typically, babies have developed a palmar grasp by about 6 months of age, although babies all develop at different rates. The palmar grasp enables them to pick up larger pieces of food in their fists and bring them up to their mouths. Foods offered to a baby using a palmar grasp need to be longer than the baby's fist, because the baby cannot access the portion of food grasped inside the fist. While your baby uses a palmar grasp, offer soft-textured foods in long strips that can be easily mashed between your thumb and forefinger. In her excellent book, *Baby-Led Feeding*, Jenna Helwig suggests using an "adult pinky finger" as a benchmark visual reference for length, width, and depth. If you find that slippery foods like mango or avocado are too hard for your baby to grasp, try rolling them in something like bread crumbs, ground almond flour, or ground flaxseed to give your baby a better grip.

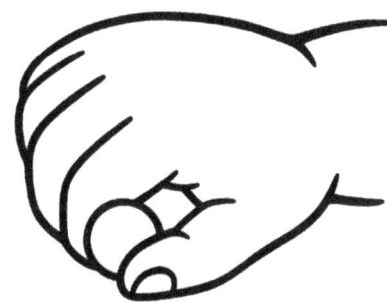

Pincer grasp: *Using the index finger and thumb to pick up an object. This important fine motor development milestone requires coordination of both the brain and muscles.*

The pincer grasp usually develops at around 9 months of age, but it can emerge earlier or later, typically in the window of time between 8 and 12 months. The pincer grasp enables babies to pick up smaller pieces of food between the thumb and forefinger. When you notice that your baby is starting to use a pincer grasp, you can start offering smaller finger foods about the size of a Cheerio™ or, per Helwig's suggestion, a chickpea. If your baby is 12 months or older and has not yet shown any signs of a pincer grasp, speak to your pediatrician. Lack of pincer grasp development at 1 year of age or older can affect self-feeding and may indicate a condition or delay that affects motor development. Your pediatrician may recommend interventions that can help, such as occupational therapy.

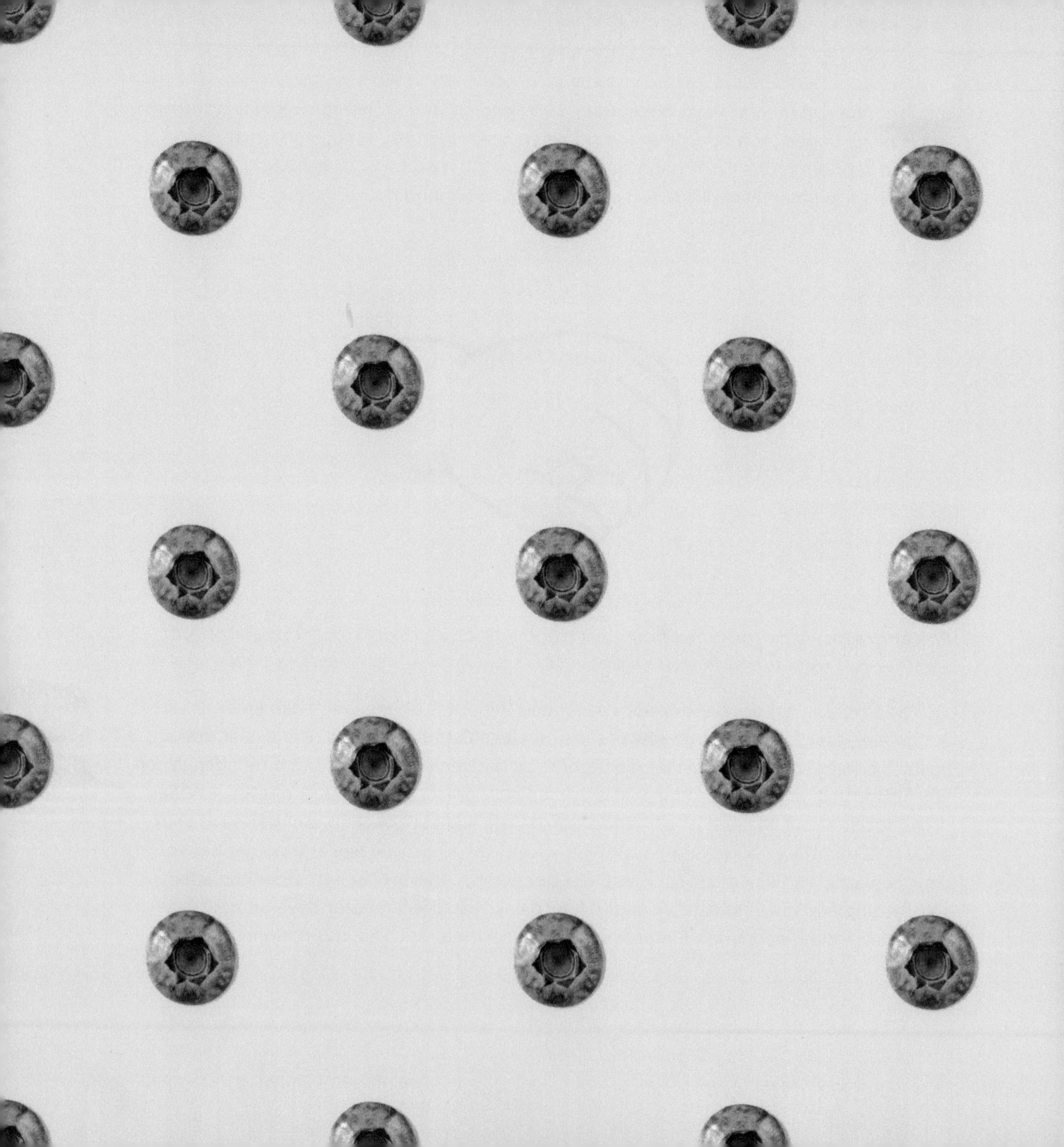

CHAPTER TWO

HERE WE GO! WHAT TO EXPECT

As you get ready to begin BLW, familiarize yourself with your role in responsive feeding. You decide when and where meals happen and what foods are offered. Unlike spoon-feeding, the key is allowing your baby to control whether to eat and how much to eat.

You may find that your baby refuses certain foods, spits out others, and makes some funny and adorable faces while experiencing new flavors. This is all normal. Resist the urge to assume any of this means your baby does not like a food, as food preferences are not a part of this stage and will develop later. Speaking of facial expressions, keep your own reactions to foods positive. Babies learn by mimicking and will be influenced by the faces you make during mealtimes.

At this early stage, it is completely normal if your baby does not end up eating much. The first few weeks of solids are more about playing than eating, and it is okay if more food ends up on the floor than in your baby's tummy. Breastfeeding or formula feeding will still be the main source of nutrition for now, which makes it easier to relax when you are not sure if mealtime is over. Some babies will communicate that they are done by shaking their heads or handing back pieces of food. Others will drop or throw food purposefully, although many do this during the first few weeks of BLW anyway. The most important thing is to read your baby's cues for fullness as best as you can and do not stress about ending the meal when the baby seems finished.

Breast Milk or Formula and Finger Foods: A Balancing Act

Even after starting solids, your baby will ideally continue to breastfeed on demand or take breast milk or formula on a regular schedule with meals in between. Feel free to offer your baby finger foods every time the family sits down to eat if it works for you, but do not worry about missing a meal if your baby is tired. The timing of the actual meals is less important than your sitting down and eating them with your baby.

A typical BLW meal schedule includes one or two meals per day (and about four milk feedings) for 6- to 7-month-olds, three meals per day for 9- to 11-month-olds, and three meals plus two snacks per day for 11+-month-olds, although every baby's needs are unique. Over time, your baby will gradually drink less breast milk or formula and eat more food, but the progression through this stage occurs according to each child's individual needs. Let your baby be the guide. As your baby's self-feeding skills improve, the amount of food consumed will also increase.

Your Baby's Palate

A common misconception about transitioning babies from 100 percent breast milk or formula to meals that incorporate solid foods is that the food offered should all be bland, which leads many parents to offer refined, processed, carbohydrate-type foods.

According to the American Academy of Pediatrics, research suggests that it is important to expose babies to a wide variety of flavors and textures early on, as this may positively influence their later food preferences and reduce the likelihood of picky eating. Although I would not recommend offering a preloaded spoon of your spiciest chili as a first food, do not be afraid to offer foods with flavor. If your baby chooses not to eat a new food you have introduced, do not assume they do not like it. Studies also show that it can take multiple repeated exposures before a child will accept a new food, so keep trying. Throughout the process, keep offering healthy foods and resist the urge to pressure, cajole, or trick your baby into taking a bite, which tends to backfire in the long run.

This stage of discovery and exploration is a good time to offer as many healthy, minimally processed whole foods as possible. The more chances babies have now to become familiar with foods that promote health (such as whole grains, beans, legumes, vegetables, fruits, nuts, and seeds), the more likely they will be to eat them in later years.

Giving Your Baby a Seat at the Family Table

Although the immediate purpose of BLW is to introduce your baby to solid foods, its core components (such as developing your baby's palate and including your baby in family meals) have a more far-reaching purpose: to put your child on a path of lifelong health and wellness. That said, the practical side of carving out time to eat together can be challenging in the context of a fast-paced family life. I have always found that when my family schedule gets crazy and I am tempted to skip the effort of making and serving family meals, it helps to be reminded of why it is so smart to make them a priority as often as possible.

Family meals offer enormous benefits for you and your baby. You will save time, money, and energy by cooking one meal for the entire family. You will avoid the expense of buying jarred baby food—or the time and effort of puréeing baby food in a blender and freezing it in ice cube trays. Your baby will benefit from the role modeling you and other family members provide at the family table, as well as the exposure to a variety of foods.

As your baby grows into a toddler, child, and teenager, the benefits of family meals expand and multiply into even more holistic areas of overall health. In 2011, the American Academy of Pediatrics published an analysis of a wide range of studies on family meals and found that kids and teens who participated in family dinners three or more times per week experienced the following positive health outcomes:

- A greater likelihood of eating and choosing healthy, nutrient-dense foods
- A reduced likelihood of being overweight
- A significantly reduced likelihood (about 35 percent) of engaging in disordered eating
- Better academic performance
- A reduced likelihood of engaging in risky behaviors (drugs, alcohol, sexual activity)
- Better relationships with parents
- Fewer emotional and behavioral problems

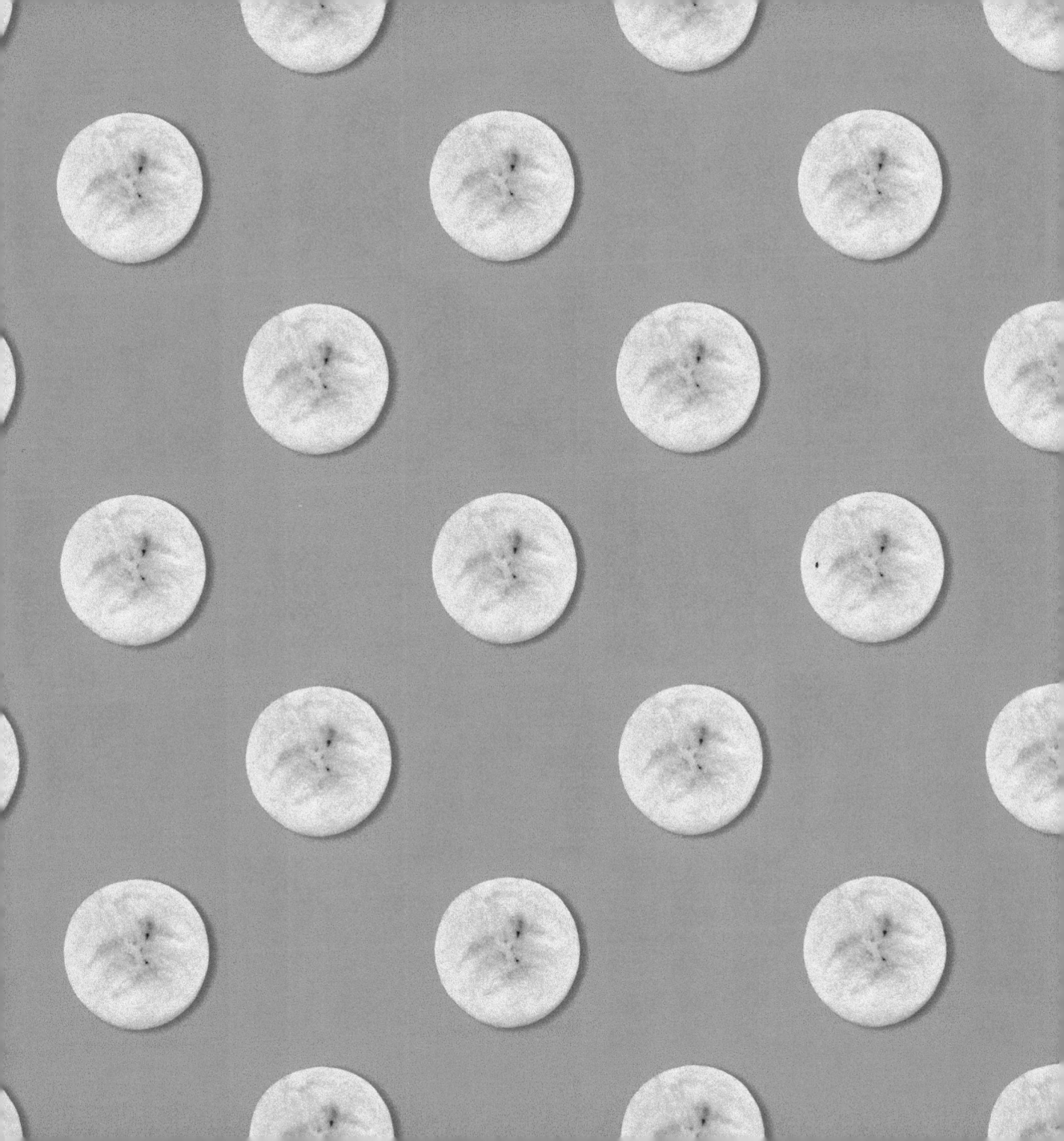

Ten Tips for Successful BLW Meals

1. **Keep mealtimes positive.**

    Time meals for when your baby is not too hungry, full, or tired. Right after breast-feeding or formula works well for some, whereas for others, it is better to wait a bit. Find what works best for your baby.

2. **Wash your baby's hands.**

    Wash yours, too!

3. **Seat your baby safely.**

    Always seat your baby upright in a high chair, with hips and knees bent at 90-degree angles. Make sure your baby is not leaning back, which increases the risk of choking. Use a high chair with foot support so your baby's feet are not dangling. Fasten the safety straps and then attach the high-chair tray, or pull the chair close to the table.

4. **Safety-test the temperature and texture of finger foods.**

    Warmed foods should feel lukewarm, not hot. Be sure that the foods are either soft enough to easily squish between your fingers (like a steamed soft stick of carrot) or large and fibrous enough not to break off into pieces when sucked (like a strip of steak). Do not offer foods that will form crumbs in the baby's mouth.

5. **Offer appropriate portions.**

    Place three or four pieces of appropriately sized finger foods on your baby's plate—not so few that your baby gets bored and not so many that it is intimidating.

6. **Always supervise mealtimes.**

    Sit with your baby and **watch closely at all times during meals**. Important safety tips: **Never leave your baby unattended with finger foods**, and **never put food in your baby's mouth**—both of these increase choking risk.

7. **Eat together as often as you can.**

Remove distractions like televisions and phones, and eat together as a family as often as your schedule allows. If family meals are not possible, try to have at least one person eat the same foods as your baby at each meal. Role modeling is a powerful and important part of the process.

8. **Offer your baby water.**

Using a small, automatic-sealing–valve, open, or straw-type cup, offer water only at mealtimes so that it does not replace breast milk or formula between meals. Skip sippy cups, which can delay oral-motor development. (Juice is not recommended for babies under 1 year, and many pediatricians and dietitians do not recommend juice at all, regardless of age.)

9. **Check for chipmunk cheeks.**

Some babies occasionally pocket pieces of food in their cheeks. Offering only a few pieces of food at a time can help prevent overstuffing of the mouth. At the end of meals, model a wide-open mouth so that your baby will also open up and allow you to check for pocketed food. If food is present, encourage your baby to drink a few sips of water, chew, and wash it down. If this is unsuccessful, you may need to carefully finger-sweep the inside of your baby's cheeks to pull the food forward and out of the mouth (be cautious not to push the food back toward the throat).

10. **Make accommodations when necessary.**

If your baby has a cold or other illness, offer breast milk or formula more often and do not worry about offering solids.

Embracing the Mess

Allowing your baby to explore the textures, colors, flavors, and smells of different foods is just as important as balancing breast milk or formula with solids, developing your baby's palate, and making time for family meals. Experiencing food as a sensory feast teaches babies to enjoy eating and helps form the foundation of a healthy relationship with food going forward. For some babies, this smashing, squishing, rolling, dropping, and throwing food is all that happens for a while. This certainly can lead to some messes at first. The reality is that feeding babies is messy no matter what approach you take, but you can still do a few things to manage it and reduce the stress:

- Invest in a high chair that promotes good, upright posture and prevents slumping, leaning back, and pulling up of the knees. The chair should have a footrest so that your baby's feet are firmly planted when the baby is seated, and it should position your baby's hips so that they face forward. I also highly recommend choosing a high chair that is easy to clean. You will thank yourself later for choosing an easy-wipe design and skipping any cushions or padding. Ideally, skip the tray as well and pull the high chair right up to the family table during meals so that your baby can see everyone and watch how they eat. My favorite high chair is the Stokke Tripp Trapp, which is definitely an investment but one that meets all the criteria, and it can be used for years as your baby grows into toddlerhood and beyond.
- Buy a few catch-all silicone bibs with a front pocket and an adjustable hook or clasp. I used to toss these bibs right into the dishwasher after meals. They should be flexible enough to be comfortable but sturdy enough to catch falling food.
- Invest in silicone plates and bowls with suction bases so that they stay put. I also like the type that have a front lip to help catch falling food. Sectioned silicone mats also help babies get a better grip on foods as they self-feed.
- Buy some baby spoons that have stainless-steel spoon parts and wide plastic or silicone handles for easier baby gripping. Silicone spoons are also fine—just be careful about letting a teething baby chew on these as they can scratch and tear easily.

- Keep a few small stainless-steel open cups on hand and WOW-style, Munchkin 360, or straw cups. (Skip the sippy cups, which can delay speech and oral-motor development.)
- Make sure you have paper towels and baby wipes for quick clean-up. Better yet, I love the more environmentally friendly option of filling an empty wipes container with small cloth wipes and a little water mixed with some castile soap; you can wash and reuse these cloths as needed.
- Keep a small handheld vacuum nearby.
- If it is warm enough, dress your baby in only a diaper and bib for mealtimes, which makes for an easy transition from the high chair to the tub.

Baby-Led Feeding Outside the Home

Hitting the road and eating out with your littlest eater can feel challenging at first, but with a bit of practice it gets easier. Being prepared helps! I would not leave home without wipes, which make clean-up exponentially easier when you are out and about. Pack a bib, an easy-wipe silicone placemat, and your baby's preferred type of non-sippy travel cup.

Here are some on-the-go snacks that work well:

- Bananas
- Avocado slices (keep the skin on each slice during your travels so that the slices hold their shape, remove the skin right before serving, and pack a small bag of ground flaxseed or bread crumbs to roll the slices in so your baby can get a good grip)
- Pancakes (make a big batch on the weekend and freeze the extras so you can toss them in your bag as a portable snack option)
- Whole-grain, low-sugar cereal or berries in a lidded snack cup (to help control spills)

Most restaurants provide high chairs and offer at least a few menu options that work well during BLW. Here are some ideas:

- Sweet potato fries
- Steamed or mashed veggies
- Meat or fish patties
- Pasta
- Scrambled eggs or omelets
- Whole-grain toast
- Pancakes
- Tomato slices
- Hummus
- Pita bread

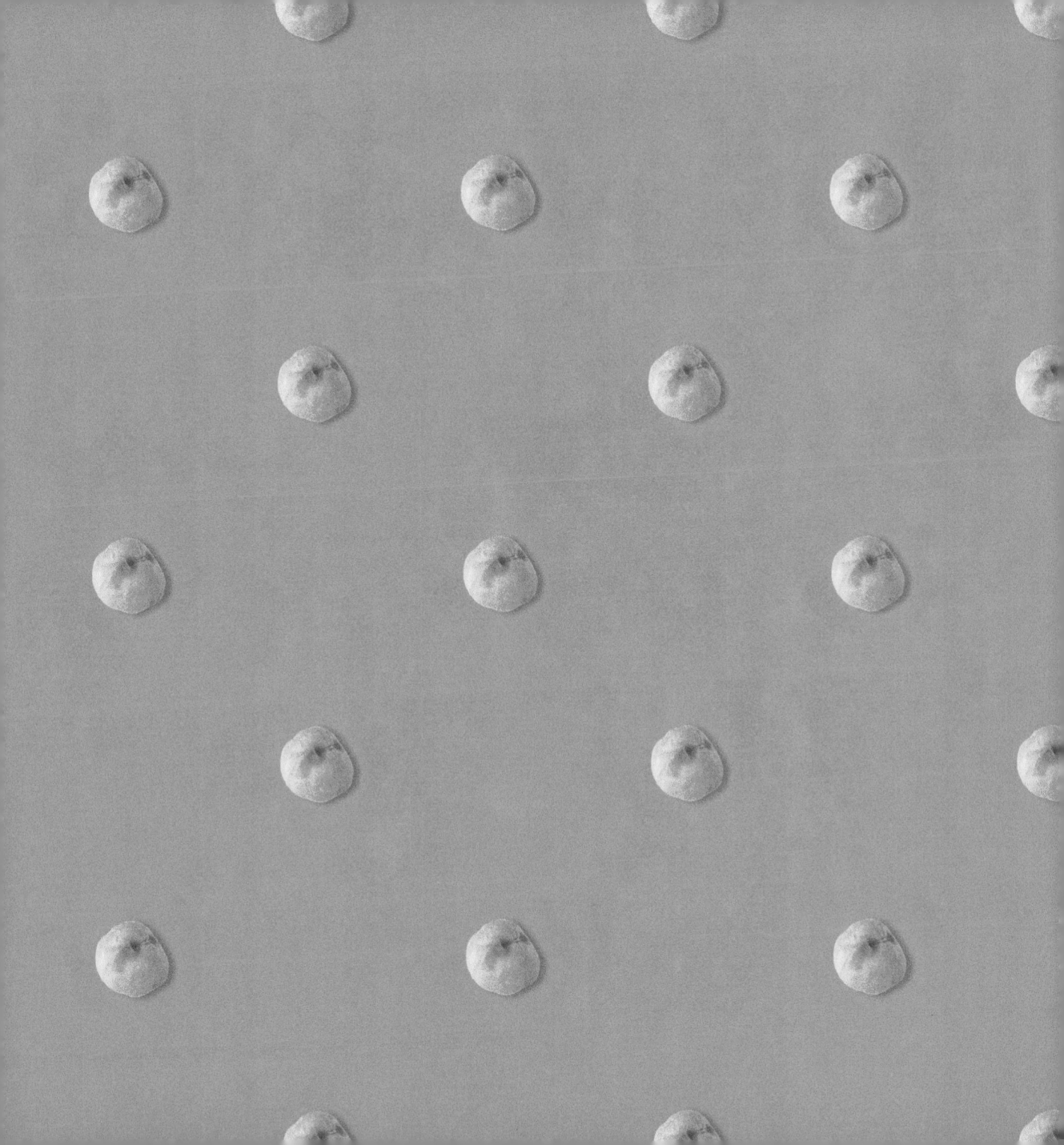

PART TWO

A PRACTICAL GUIDE TO SAFE & HEALTHY BABY-LED WEANING

Despite the fact that BLW has been growing steadily in popularity among dietitians, pediatricians, and pediatric feeding experts, many parents lack the confidence in their own ability to appropriately size food and reduce choking risk when preparing first foods for their babies. The overall goal of the second part of this book is to reduce stress and bolster your confidence by providing specific answers to all the granular questions you might have about how to safely prepare first foods.

When I say specific, I mean detailed descriptions and unambiguous, to-scale visual references about how to prepare your baby's food, how to recognize the difference between gagging and choking and what to do about each, how to combine different types of foods to meet your baby's nutrition needs, which specific foods are best to start with, and which foods should be avoided. All of this is accompanied by information about specific, important nutrients and answers to questions about vegetarianism, organic foods, and more.

CHAPTER THREE

BITE-SIZING BASICS

onfidence begins with knowledge. Being able to recognize your baby's developmental stage, understanding the role of texture, and knowing how to cook, cut, and offer first foods to your baby will go a long way toward building your confidence with BLW. Through it all, remember that you know your baby best.

Keeping your baby safe is of topmost priority, so it is important to observe and note your child's development as you progress through BLW—from the introduction of solids until your baby has teeth and can chew and swallow OR chew and spit out foods. The timeline of this progression is different from baby to baby, but it generally occurs between about 6 and 12 months of age. During the time that your baby has few (if any) teeth and cannot chew and swallow or chew and spit out a food, you should offer only foods that are very soft and tender. Over time, as you notice your baby's self-feeding skills developing, you can gradually introduce slightly harder foods that can still be easily gummed.

Here are some guidelines:

- In general, until your baby can chew and swallow or chew and spit out foods, **avoid crumbly foods or foods that break into crumbs in the mouth, like dry crackers. Also avoid any hard foods that can split off easily into pieces, as well as any hard, coin-shaped foods that are the size and shape of a windpipe**—all of these are choking hazards.
- **Make sure that foods are very soft and tender enough to easily mash between your thumb and forefinger.** This allows your baby to mash the food on the roof of the mouth before swallowing, which greatly reduces the likelihood of choking.
- While your baby uses a palmar grasp (typically until about 8 or 9 months of age), cut foods into "fingers." Fingers of soft fruits and vegetables should be about ½ inch wide by ½ inch deep by 3 inches long, or about the size of an adult pinky finger. Fingers of toast, pancakes, and French toast should be about 1 inch wide (roughly the width of two adult pinky fingers). Do not expect that your baby will

finish an entire piece of food at this stage. Most babies will be able to access only the part of the food sticking out of the closed fist. The goal of offering fingers of meats at this stage is to let your baby suck out the iron-rich juices rather than eat the meat itself—your careful supervision is especially important here.

- When your baby develops a pincer grasp—typically at around 8 or 9 months—you can start offering soft, easily mashed foods that are roughly the size of a chickpea. At this stage, you can also continue to offer larger pieces of tender foods like omelet or avocado, but avoid the larger, finger-size meats that can become choking hazards once your baby can rip off smaller pieces from a strip. Instead, cut these meats into small, chickpea-size bites.

- You might be wondering whether foods with a puréed texture, like yogurt or applesauce, are allowed during BLW. Purées are simply a texture, like any other. The more important consideration is whether your baby is being given the chance to choose whether and how much to eat. There is no research that suggests that a combined approach of offering both finger foods and purées increases choking risk. If you find that offering more purées along with finger foods works better for your baby and reduces your own stress levels, feel free to offer a combination. You can offer purées the BLW way—by serving them on a preloaded spoon or letting your baby scoop them up by hand (either way, just make sure that your baby is self-feeding). If the purée does not stay on the spoon, try mixing in a little iron-fortified baby cereal, which helps thicken the consistency while boosting iron intake.

- Trust your gut. If you have noticed that a certain food seems to cause more gagging or makes you nervous, skip it and come back to it a few weeks later when your baby's self-feeding skills have developed further.

Gagging and Choking: Learn to Spot the Difference

For a baby, learning to eat finger foods is a brand-new experience that involves chewing, swallowing, and breathing all at the same time. Depending on the texture of the food offered, a 6- or 7-month-old baby may gag often (and more so at first than a spoon-fed baby). Gagging, not to be confused with choking, is a noisy, normal, built-in safety mechanism that can sound disturbing but is nothing more than the process of coughing and bringing up food that the baby is not ready to swallow.

Early on, the gag reflex is strong. Over time, it shifts further back into the mouth and by around the age of 9 months, it becomes similar to an adult gag reflex and subsides. During a moment of gagging, you can help your baby by staying calm and positive and encouraging chewing.

On the other hand, choking is a silent, serious event that happens when a larger piece of food gets lodged in the airway and blocks it. The baby may become distressed, turn blue, and grab at the throat, but no air is passing through it. Intervention is usually needed to force the food out of the baby's airway.

Recent studies have found that BLW is not associated with an increased risk of choking. In fact, a 2017 study published in the *Journal of Human Nutrition and Dietetics* found that babies who were offered finger foods the least often had the highest frequency of choking episodes, and a 2016 study in *Pediatrics* found that by the time they reach the age of 8 months, BLW infants gag less frequently than their spoon-fed counterparts. Still, parents and caregivers should be well-informed, take a training course and become certified in infant first aid and CPR, and make every effort to proceed safely.

The best defense against choking is knowing which foods are choking hazards, avoiding them, and offering only finger foods that have been prepared in a safe, appropriate manner.

Choking 101

Even after hearing about research suggesting that choking during BLW is much less likely than you would think, most parents, grandparents, and caregivers will tell you that the biggest barrier they have to BLW is the fear of choking. When my girls were babies, I remember being surprised by my own very calm, laid-back mother panicking whenever my girls would start to gag or cough on a bite of food.

If the idea, sound, and sight of a baby gagging makes you nervous, you are not alone. Take comfort in the knowledge that no matter which feeding method you choose, learning to eat is a skill that babies need to develop over time and with practice. Learning to eat can be scary, but it is an inevitable part of growth. The good news about BLW is that a BLW infant has earlier and more frequent chances to practice, hone, and improve these skills.

One way to reduce any stress you might have about choking is to educate yourself and anyone else who may be caring for your baby on the difference between gagging and choking and what to do should your baby start to choke on a piece of food or any other object. This is crucial safety information for *all* caregivers, whether or not BLW is in the mix! Most importantly—do not panic. Stay calm and focused so that you can provide the care your baby needs.

Familiarize yourself with the steps involved in responding to a choking emergency:

- In the event of a choking emergency, remember to stay calm.
- Note whether your baby is coughing forcefully or crying hard. If the answer is yes to either, do not administer first aid. Both forceful coughing and strong crying indicate that the airway is not blocked. If any object or piece of food is partially blocking the airway, coughing and crying can help push it out.
- If your baby's skin is turning a bluish color or if your baby is struggling to breathe and unable to cry, call 911 and administer first aid.
- Sit down and lay your baby face-down along your nondominant forearm, using your thighs for support.

- Firmly and securely hold the baby's jaw with the thumb and fingers of your non-dominant hand, then tip your baby's head down so that it is lower than its torso.
- In the space between your baby's shoulder blades, deliver five firm, quick blows using the heel of your dominant hand.
- If after five blows, the object does not dislodge, turn the baby face-up along your lap, supporting the head with your nondominant hand and keeping the head below its torso.
- Position two fingers in the middle of the baby's breastbone, just below its nipple line, and administer a series of five quick, smooth thrusts, compressing the breastbone about 1/2 inch.
  Repeat the five back blows and five chest thrusts until the object becomes dislodged or until the baby loses consciousness.
- If your baby has lost consciousness, shout for help, perform infant CPR for 1 minute, and then call 911 and follow the operator's instructions.
- If the baby is unconscious and you can see the object blocking the airway, try to remove it with your finger (but never try to grasp and remove an object lodged in the airway if a baby is alert).
- Always be prepared. You and any other adults who will be caring for your baby should take a training course and become certified in infant first aid and CPR. The Red Cross (www.redcross.org) offers an accredited and affordable online Child and Baby First Aid/CPR/AED course that you can take anytime, anywhere.

Smart and Safe Kitchen Habits

Another concern for those new to BLW is foodborne illness. Because it can cause symptoms such as fever, headache, diarrhea, and stomachache, many cases are likely mistaken for viruses or the flu. According to a 2011 report by the Centers for Disease Control and Prevention, an estimated one in six Americans get sick and 128,000 are hospitalized each year as a result of foodborne illness.

The immune systems of most healthy adults can generally handle small amounts of harmful bacteria, although reactions vary from person to person and depend on many variables such as the type of bacteria and how much was eaten. Although anyone can be affected, foodborne illness is particularly dangerous for babies because their immune systems are not yet fully developed. Be sure to make these basic food safety guidelines a consistent part of your routine:

- Before you prepare or handle any food, wash your hands with soap under warm running water for at least 20 seconds. Always wash them again after handling any raw eggs or raw meats.
- Defrost foods safely overnight in the refrigerator—not on countertops or in the sink! If you plan to cook the food immediately, defrosting in the microwave is okay.
- Avoid cross-contamination by using one cutting board for produce and a separate cutting board for meat, poultry, and fish; thoroughly wash and disinfect all cutting boards, surfaces, and utensils before using them again, especially those that come in contact with raw meat and raw eggs.
- When in doubt, throw it out!
- Keep cold foods cold and hot foods hot. The temperature danger zone for most foods is between 40 and 140 degrees Fahrenheit (4.44 degrees and 60 degrees Celsius). Foods that remain in this zone for more than 4 hours can start harboring pathogenic microorganisms and should be discarded. Leftovers kept at room temperature for more than 2 hours should be tossed as well.
- Wash fruits and vegetables thoroughly before prepping, even if you do not plan on eating the skin. This is so that nothing from the outside contaminates the inside flesh during peeling and slicing.
- Using a dial or digital food thermometer, prepare protein foods according to the USDA's Safe Minimum Internal Temperature Chart for beef, veal, pork, and lamb steaks and roasts (145 degrees Fahrenheit or 62.8 degrees Celsius); hamburger and egg dishes (160 degrees Fahrenheit or 71.1 degrees Celsius); and all poultry (165 degrees Fahrenheit or 73.9 degrees Celsius).
- When you reheat leftovers, bring all foods to an internal temperature of 165 degrees Fahrenheit (73.9 degrees Celsius).

Safer Serving and Storing

Some chemicals in the plastics, glues, dyes, and coatings used in food packaging, including storage containers, dishes, and utensils, may pose a risk to babies and children. These chemicals are endocrine disruptors, which means that they interrupt the normal functioning of hormones. This can lead to negative effects such as an increased risk of obesity and attention-deficit/hyperactivity disorder (ADHD) symptoms, a change in the timing and effect of puberty, and other gastrointestinal and metabolic health issues.

As a result, the American Academy of Pediatrics recommends that you do not microwave food and beverages in plastic or put plastics in the dishwasher; instead, stock your kitchen with alternatives to plastic, such as stainless steel or glass. If possible, avoid plastics with the recycling codes 3, 6, and 7 altogether. You can further reduce your baby's risk by choosing feeding plates, cups, and utensils made from stainless steel, silicone, or bamboo, and storing any leftover foods in glass containers rather than plastic ones.

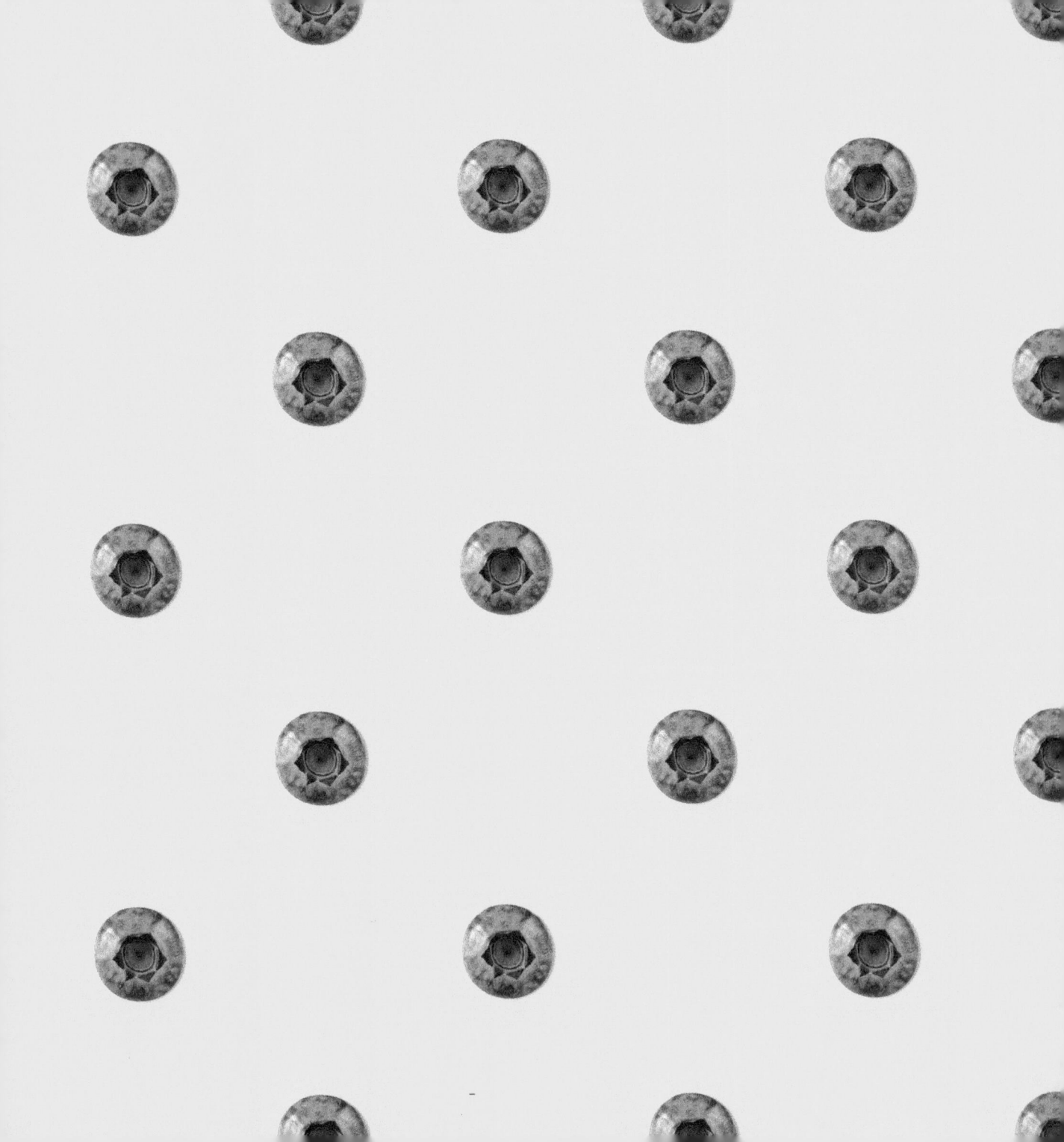

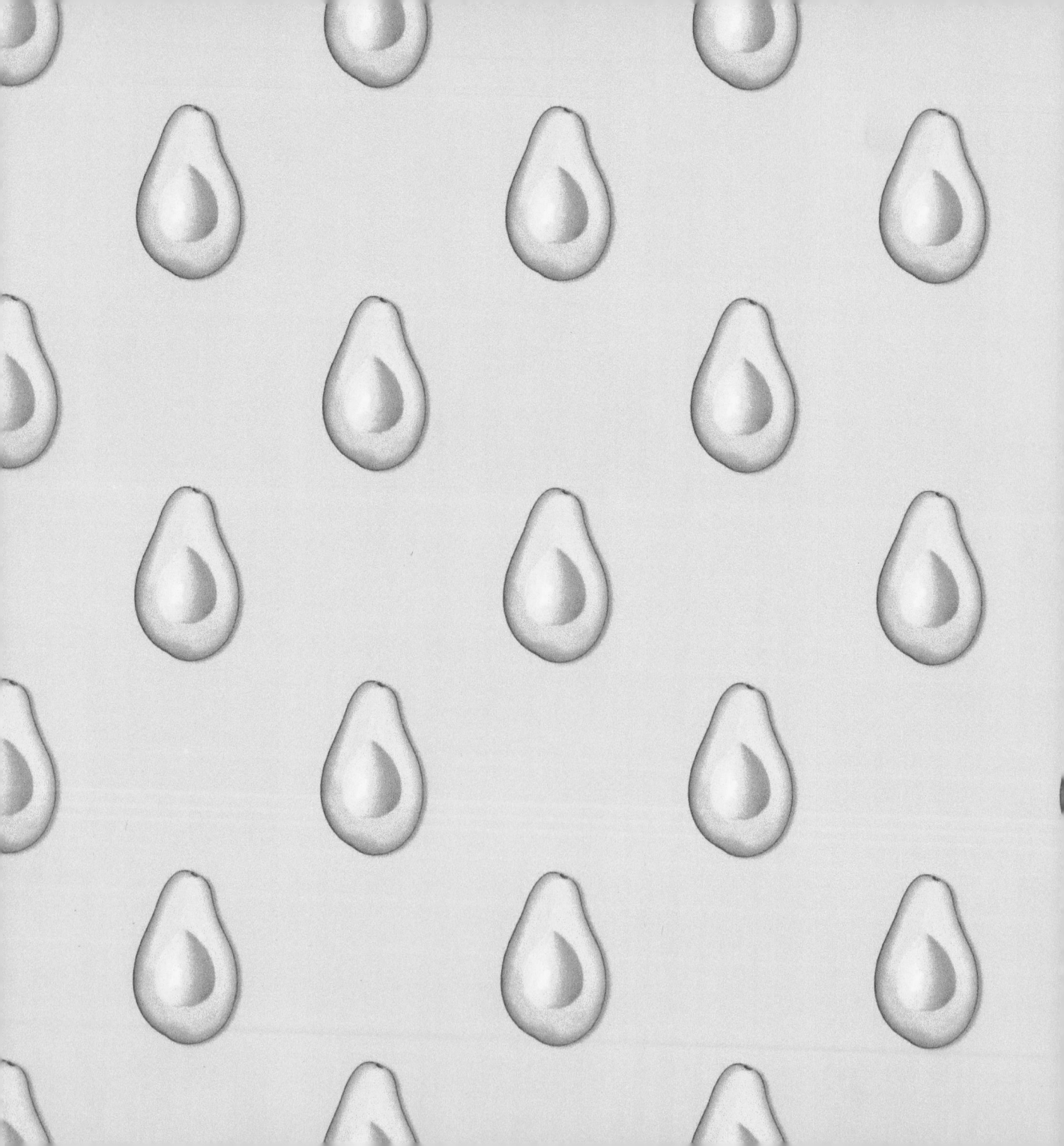

CHAPTER FOUR

BUILDING A BALANCED BABY MEAL

ontinuing to offer breast milk or formula throughout the first year of life is an essential way to ensure that your baby's nutritional needs are being met. It will become increasingly important as your baby progresses through BLW to prepare meals made from a combination of foods that provide the greatest nutritional benefit. Have you heard the phrase "Food before one is just for fun?" It gets thrown around often in online parenting communities and forums, likely as a way of encouraging longer breastfeeding, but it is not the case. Although the fun factor is certainly important, food during that first year also needs to contribute to your baby's nutritional needs, particularly for iron.

The next section will walk you through how to prepare 26 excellent first foods for babies and combine them into meals. Per the 2015 BLISS study published in *BMC Pediatrics*, these foods are divided into three groups:

- Iron-rich protein foods
- Fruits and vegetables rich in vitamin C
- Energy-rich foods

To build nutrient-dense, balanced meals for your baby, simply choose one food from each group at meals, occasionally adding a fourth food to balance out the plate. Here are some examples:

BREAKFAST 1

- Hard-boiled egg (iron/protein food), mango slices (fruit or vegetable rich in vitamin C), and pancake fingers (energy food)

BREAKFAST 2

- French toast fingers (energy and iron/protein foods), mandarin orange slices (fruit or vegetable rich in vitamin C), and yogurt (energy food)

LUNCH 1

- Toast fingers spread with hummus (energy and iron/protein foods), strawberries (fruit or vegetable rich in vitamin C), and steamed green beans (vegetable)

LUNCH 2

- Lentil and sweet potato stew (iron/protein food), kiwi slices (fruit or vegetable rich in vitamin C), and avocado slices (energy food) rolled in hemp hearts or ground flaxseed (iron/protein food)

DINNER 1

- Chickpea penne pasta (iron/protein and energy food), tomato sauce (fruit or vegetable rich in vitamin C), grated Parmesan cheese (energy food), and steamed asparagus spears (vegetable)

DINNER 2

- Baked salmon (iron/protein food), steamed broccoli (fruit or vegetable rich in vitamin C), crinkle-cut sweet potato fingers (vegetable), and buttered toast fingers (energy food)

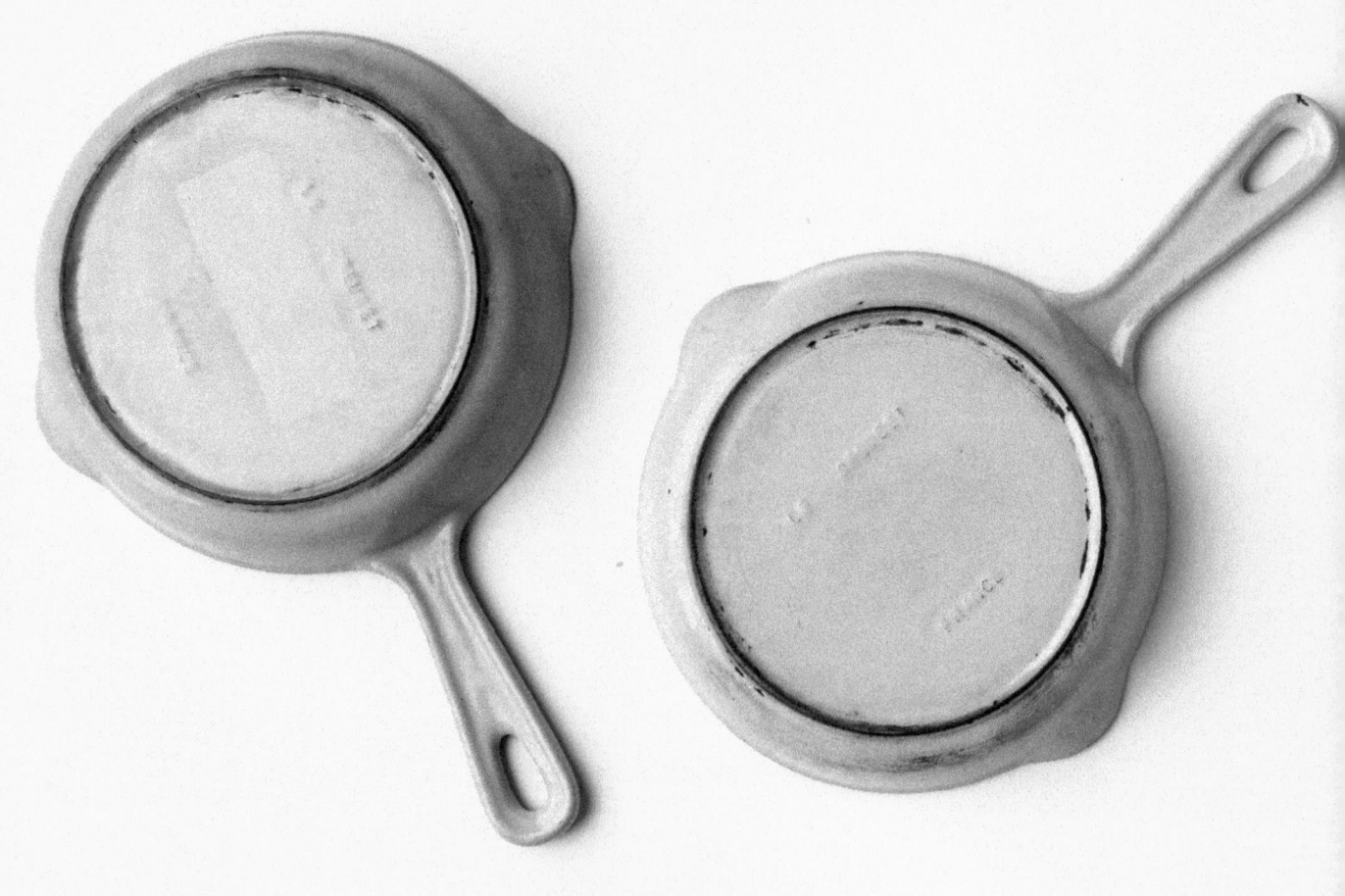

Nutrients to Note: Iron

Although breast milk or formula is the most important source of nutrition throughout your baby's first year, it is important to maximize the nutrition in every bite of food and choose first foods strategically so that your baby gets nutrients that, at this stage, may be at lower levels in the body—most notably iron.

Iron plays an important role in the formation of hemoglobin, which is the part of red blood cells that carry oxygen throughout the body. Iron is also essential for brain and immune system development, as well as overall growth.

Breast milk is low in iron, but during the last few months before birth, full-term babies accumulate enough iron stores to last throughout the first 4 to 6 months of life. Thereafter, babies need to get their iron from food sources. This is why it is important to choose iron-rich first foods as well as food combinations that maximize iron absorption when starting solids, particularly for breastfed babies. Do not stress, though, about calculating milligrams. According to a 2018 study in *Nutrients*, you can support adequate iron intake and offer an overall balanced diet by including an iron-rich protein food, a fruit or a vegetable, and a high-energy food at each meal. Other ways to maximize your baby's iron absorption include cooking in cast iron pans, pairing iron-rich foods with vitamin C-rich foods, and adding iron-fortified baby cereal to purées and other recipes.

When in Doubt, Size it Out

If the thought of estimating food sizes for your baby using reference objects like fingers, chickpeas, or Cheerios is stressful, don't feel like you need to break out a ruler or measuring tape. I've included a diagram here, that is 100% to scale, to use as a sizing guide.

Feel free to tear it out and post it on the fridge if it will give you more confidence as you prepare food for your baby. Know that it will only get easier over time to get a sense for what sizes and shapes work best. Confidence in your baby's ability to safely self-feed will grow with each meal and snack, as your baby's feeding skills develop and improve.

Remember also that texture is just as important (if not more important) at this stage than size. If the foods offered are soft and can be easily smashed between your thumb and forefinger, the likelihood of choking goes down substantially.

Palmar

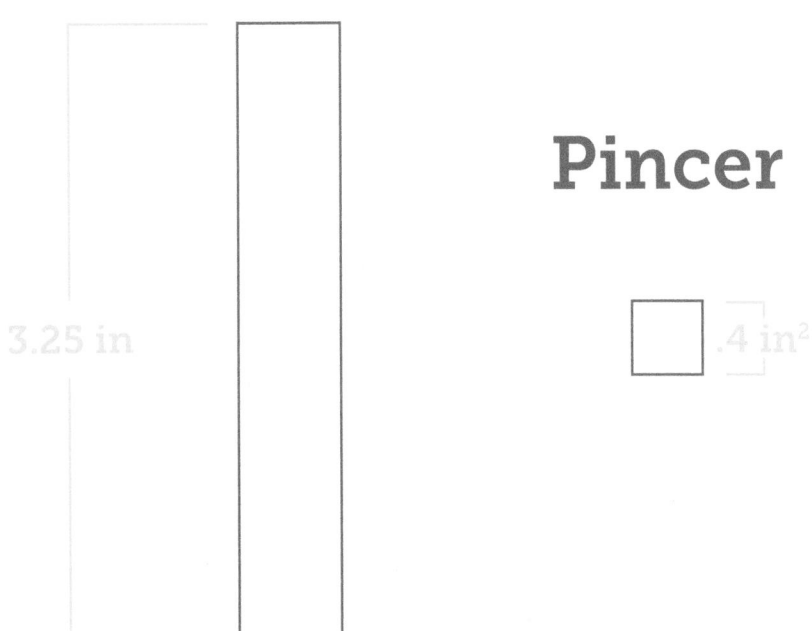

Pincer

3.25 in

.4 in²

*Don't break out the ruler! Use this instead. Diagram is at 100% scale so you can use this as a sizing reference.

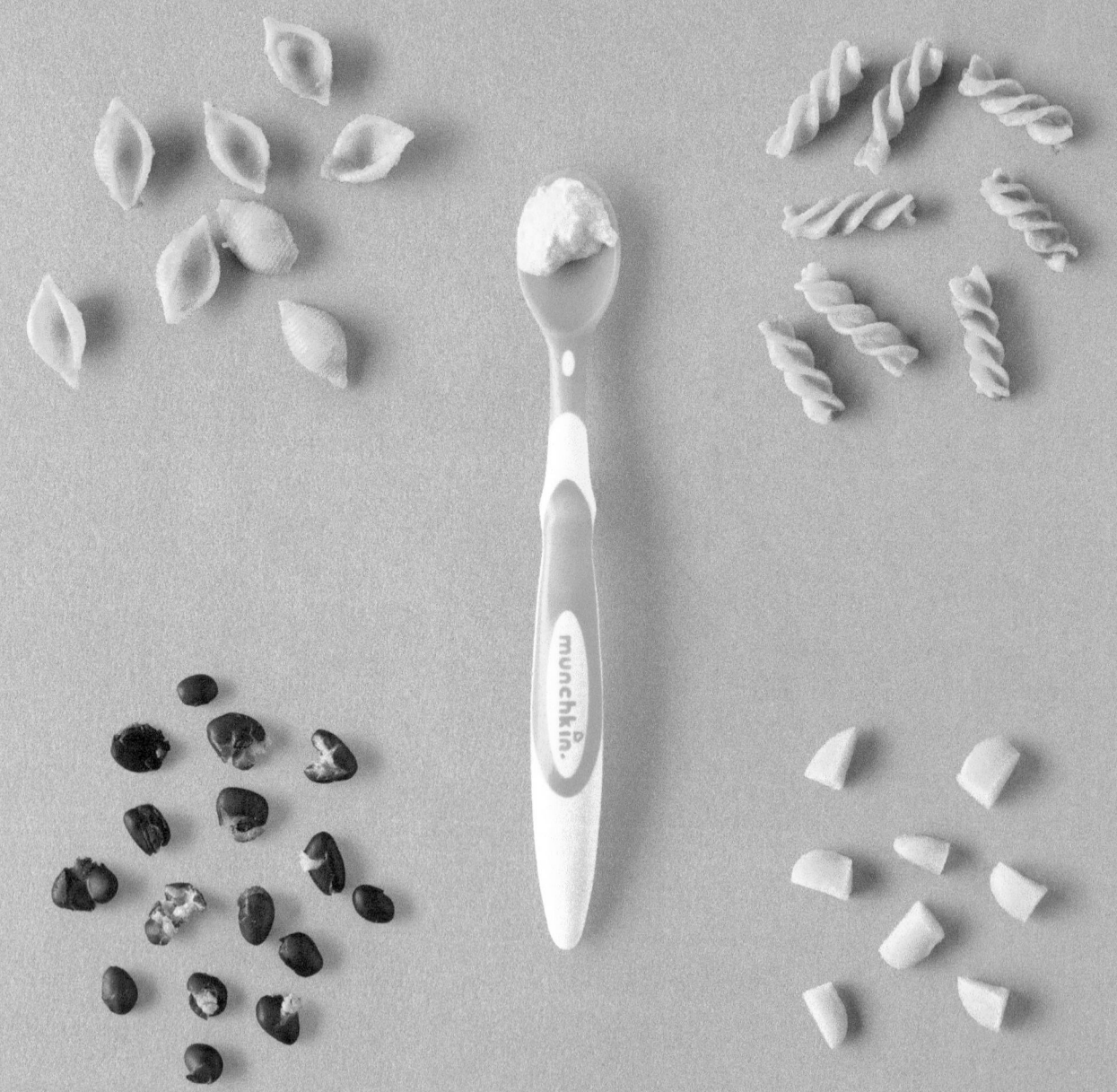

Iron-Rich Protein Foods

You can build and maintain your baby's iron levels by offering iron-rich plant- or animal-based foods. Many of these foods also contain protein, zinc, choline, and other essential vitamins and minerals that will help keep your baby healthy. I have included preparation instructions for each food based on whether your baby is using a palmar or pincer grasp.

Beans and Legumes

Rich in iron, plant-based protein, fiber, vitamins, and minerals, beans and legumes are powerhouses of convenient, affordable, tasty nutrition. Black beans, lentils, and other legumes all work well as an alternative to meat when seasoned, cooked, and formed into moist patties or balls. Try serving them a few different ways, and learn what works best for your baby.

Palmar grasp: Offer pieces of overcooked chickpea or red lentil pasta (fusilli, farfalle or bowtie, and penne shapes are often easier to grasp). You can also offer hummus or bean mash on a preloaded spoon, or let your baby use their fingers to scoop it up and into their mouth. They may also be able to grab fistfuls of well-cooked lentils or other soft, mushy legumes that stick together.

Pincer grasp: Offer soft-cooked, mashed beans. Any soft-cooked beans are great—including kidney or cannellini beans—but just be sure that they are soft and smashed, halved, or even quartered (if large) before serving. Continue offering overcooked chickpea and lentil pasta. Smaller shapes such as shells work at this stage as well. Lentil soup, bean stew, or hummus can also be served on a preloaded spoon.

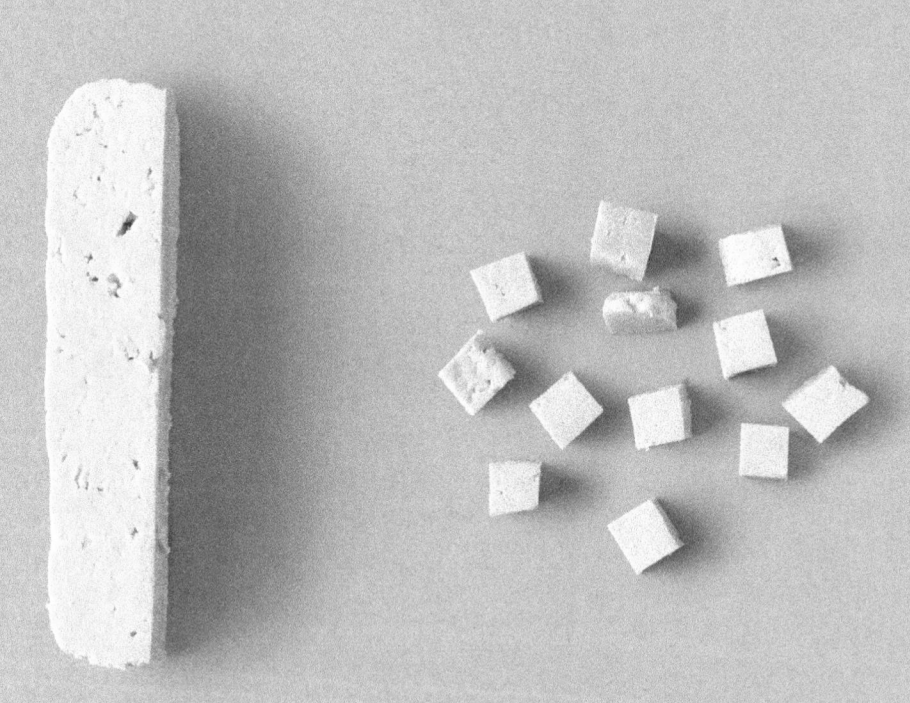

Tofu

Mild in flavor and with a great texture for babies, tofu is also a terrific source of iron and plant-based protein. Some common misconceptions about soy (based mostly on animal studies) are that it negatively affects male sex hormones and thyroid function and increases cancer risk in humans. Recent human studies published in *Fertility and Sterility,* the *Asian Pacific Journal of Cancer Prevention,* and *Thyroid* suggest neutral to positive health effects of high soy intake, so you can feel good about serving soy and soy foods to your baby. Although both firm and extra-firm versions of tofu are usually soft enough to serve to babies, check that the pieces smash easily between your thumb and forefinger before serving.

Palmar grasp: Offer adult pinky-finger-size sticks of cooked, firm, or extra-firm tofu.

Pincer grasp: Chop the tofu into chickpea-size bites.

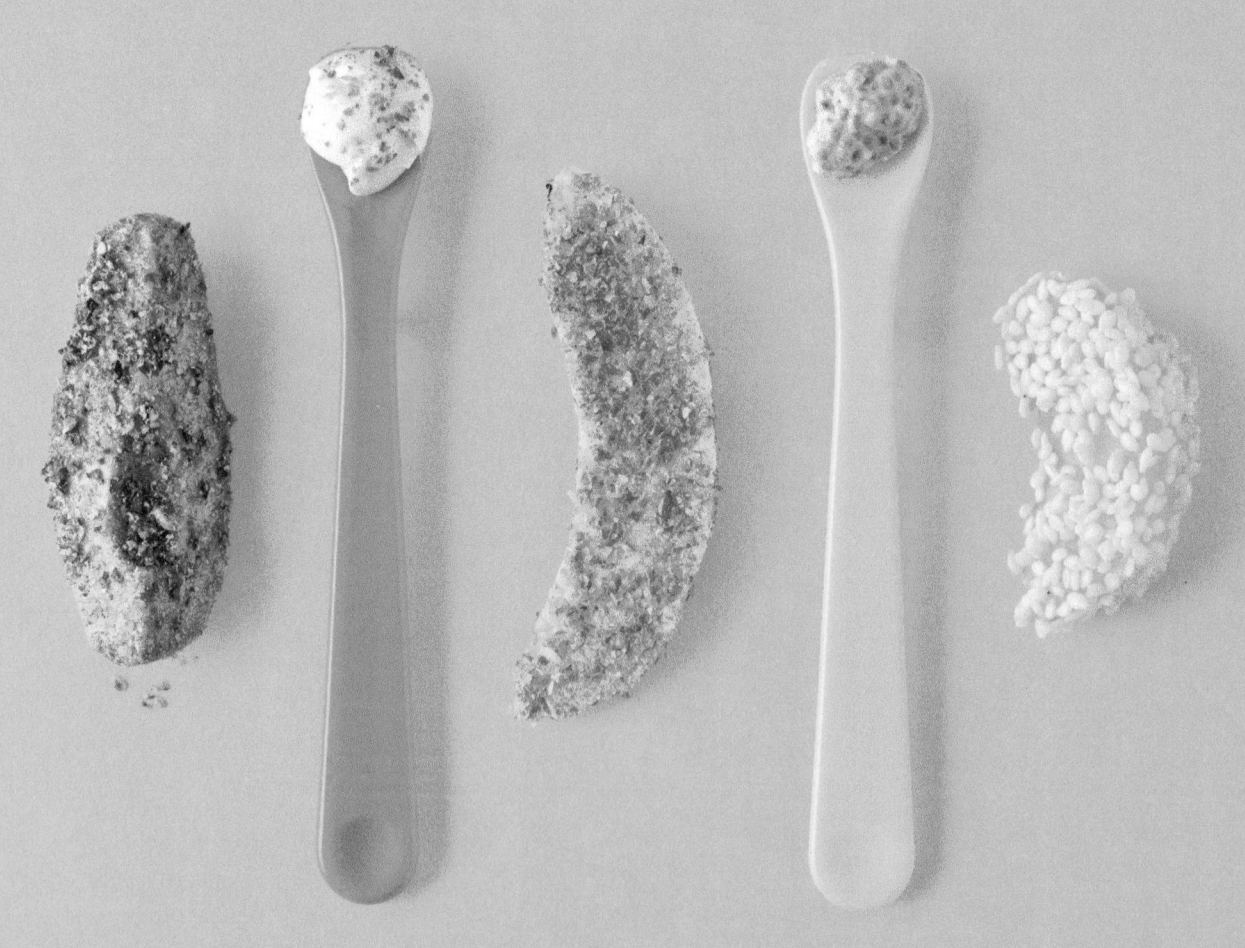

Seeds: Sesame, Hemp, Chia, and Ground Flaxseed

Seeds are nutrient-dense and bursting with protein, omega-3 fatty acids, zinc, and iron—all important nutrients for babies. You can serve these softer, small seeds to babies in many creative ways. One of my favorites is to take fingers of some of the more slippery fruits like ripe avocado, banana, plum, and mango and roll them in a teaspoon or two of hemp hearts, sesame seeds, or ground flaxseed, which helps give your baby a better grip as well as a nutrient boost. You can add them to oatmeal, yogurt, or mashed avocado, or make a chia seed pudding (especially when it is made with coconut milk for additional calories and fat) and offer it to your baby on a preloaded spoon.

Are Vegan and Vegetarian Diets Safe for Babies?

Have you ever wondered whether your baby can get all the nutrients needed from a vegan or vegetarian diet? According to the Academy of Nutrition and Dietetics, when planned appropriately, vegan and vegetarian dietary patterns can absolutely provide all the necessary nutrients needed throughout all stages of the life cycle, including infancy. Nuts, seeds, beans, legumes, and tofu are some examples of iron-rich, plant-based protein sources that with the right preparation can provide many of the nutrients your baby needs to thrive and grow.

Eight Vegan Protein and Iron Sources

- Beans
- Chickpea pasta
- Edamame
- Hummus

- Lentils
- Nuts and seeds
- Whole grains
- Tofu

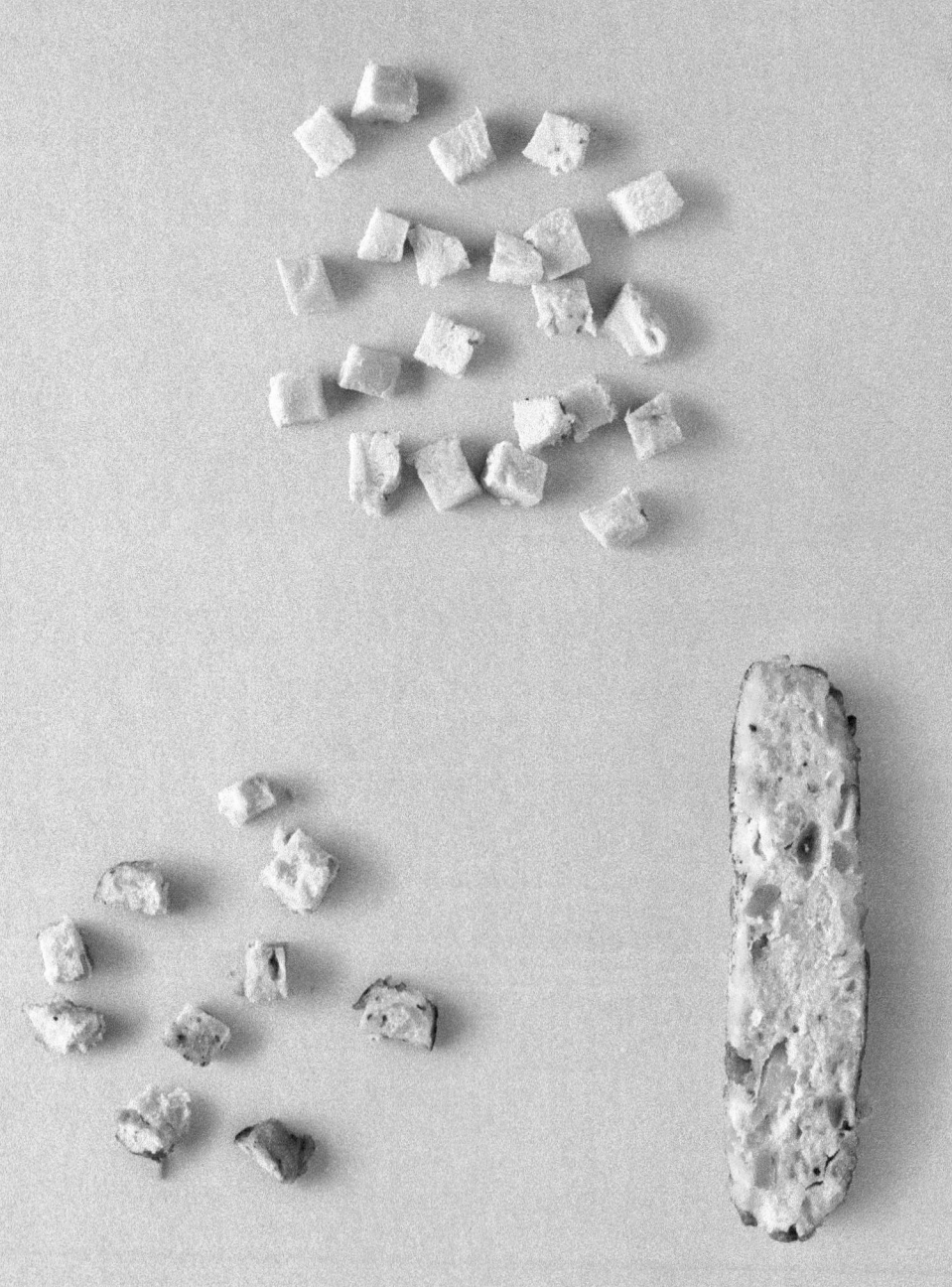

Chicken and Turkey

Iron-rich and a high-quality source of protein, chicken and turkey can be offered in a variety of ways. As long as they are cooked until very tender and the skin is removed, you can serve pieces of white or dark meat.

Palmar grasp: Shape moist, ground chicken or turkey into adult pinky-finger-size pieces that are longer than your baby's fist. Another alternative is to offer a whole drumstick, which happens to have a perfect, baby-size handle. To do so, first remove the skin, any gristle, and that thinner, pointy little bone that sits beside the larger bone. Then model how to eat it and let your baby nibble pieces right off the bone.

Pincer grasp: Cut tender-cooked chicken or turkey into bite-size pieces about the size of a chickpea, or offer it soft-shredded and moist.

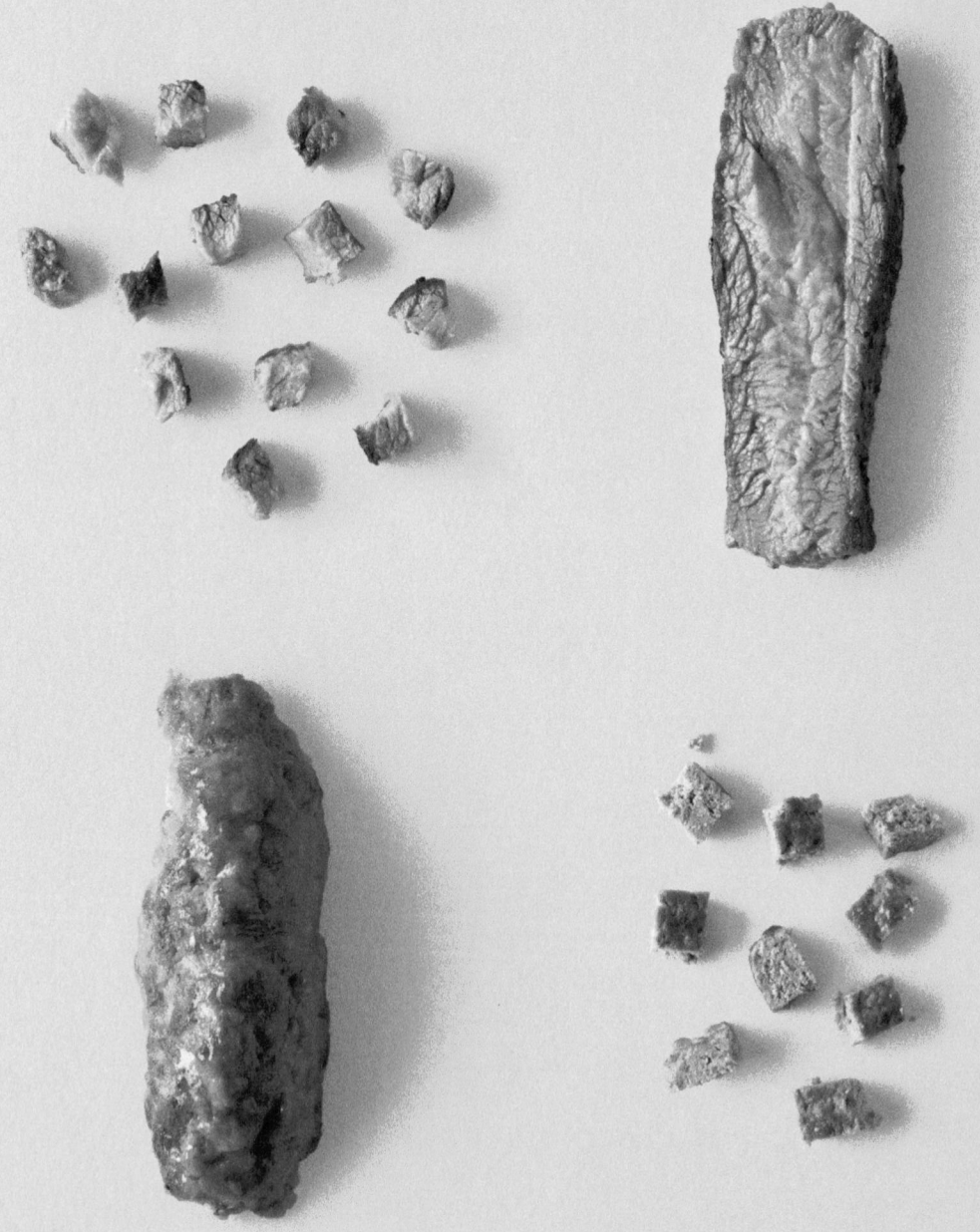

Beef

Beef is an excellent source of iron. With regard to steak, which should be cooked medium to medium-well (145 degrees Fahrenheit or 62.8 degrees Celsius), the goal in the beginning is for your baby to suck out the juices rather than eat the actual meat. On the other hand, meatballs, ground beef, and other meats and patties shaped into strips are often easier for babies to negotiate as long as they are very tender. Younger babies sometimes have an easier time swallowing ground meats that are served in a sauce.

Palmar grasp: Slice the steak against the grain into adult pinky-finger-size strips that are longer than your baby's fist. Serve one strip at a time. It is okay if a steak strip is a little wider than an adult finger as long as your baby cannot bite off a piece yet. Once your baby can bite off pieces of meat, it is time to graduate to bite-size pieces. Serve halved meatballs and tender, moist beef patties seasoned and shaped into adult finger-size strips.

Pincer grasp: Stop serving larger, finger-length strips of meat at this stage. Instead, serve tender-cooked steak cut into bite-size pieces about the size of a chickpea. Continue offering tender, moist fingers or meatballs of ground meats cut into smaller chickpea-size pieces.

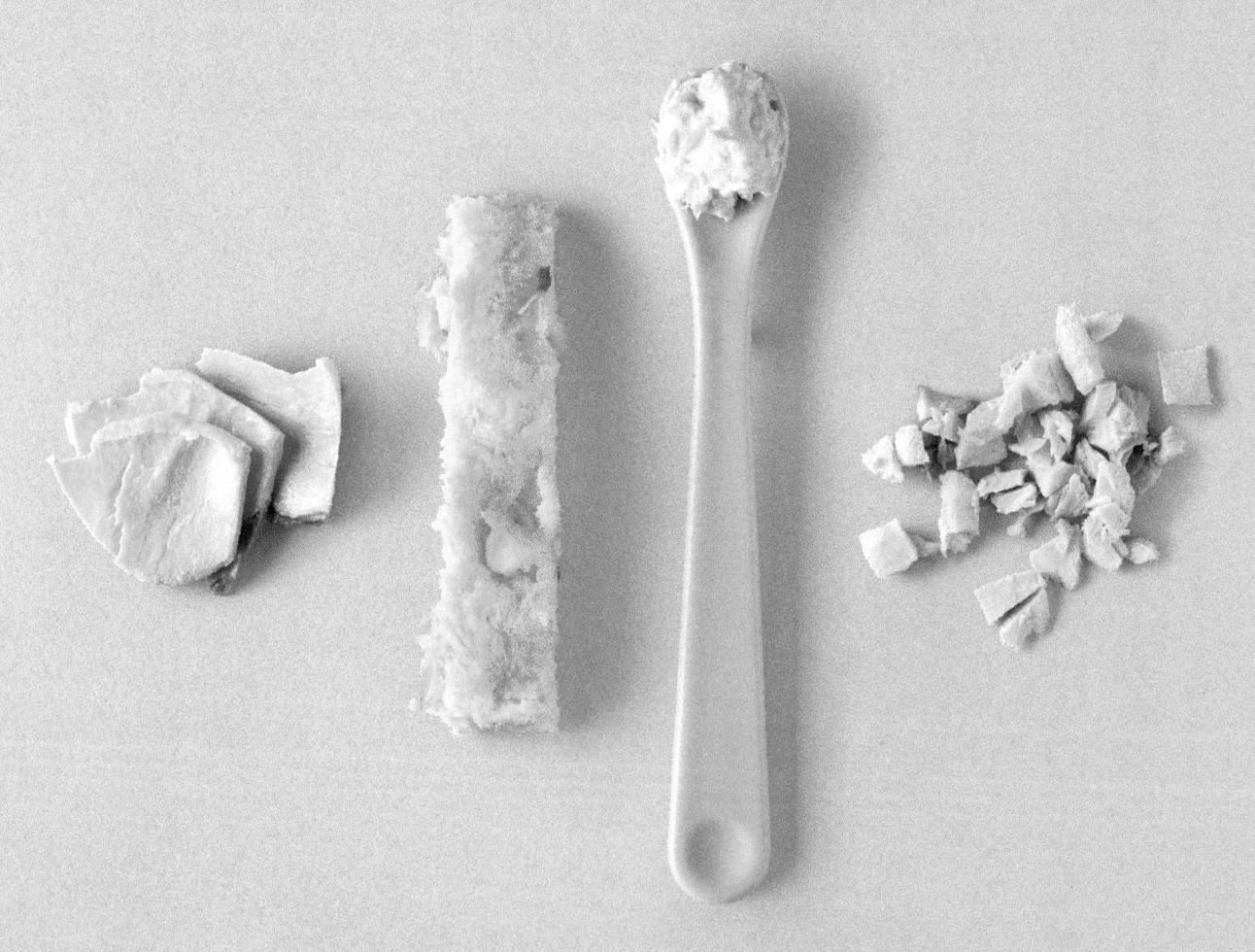

Fish

In addition to providing iron and high-quality protein, fish is a great source of omega-3 fatty acids, which play an essential role in the development of the brain, eyes, and central nervous system. If your baby is not at risk for food allergies, serve fish early and often, either one or two servings per week. Choose moist, low-mercury options like salmon, trout, pollock, herring, cod, and flounder that flake easily when cooked.

Palmar grasp: Serve pieces of cooked fish that flake easily. Be sure to remove any bones. For easier gripping, try seasoning the fish with bread crumbs or serving fish cakes cut into finger-shaped strips. If your baby has trouble gripping pieces of fish, you can try mixing it into hummus or yogurt for easier scooping with the hands.

Pincer grasp: Follow the same instructions as the beef on page 53, or cut into chickpea-size pieces.

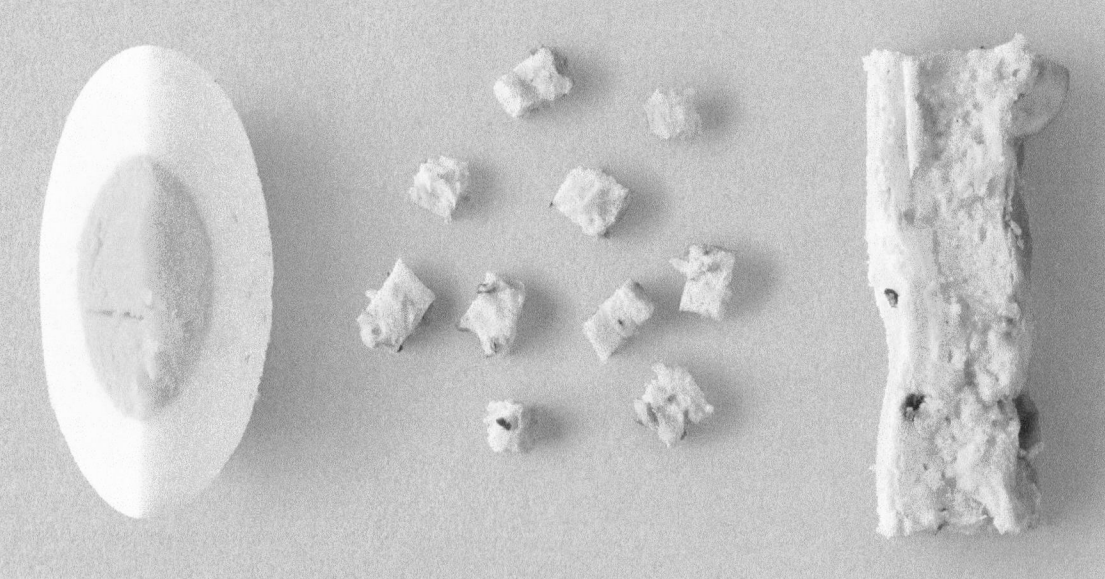

Eggs

Not only do eggs contain iron and high-quality protein, they are also an excellent source of eight essential nutrients, including lutein and choline, which are critical for proper brain development in infants and children. Look for omega-3-enriched eggs, which can also help increase your baby's intake of these essential fatty acids. Do not skip the yolk, which is where most of these nutrients are concentrated.

For safety, be sure to always cook eggs properly before serving them to your baby so that any potential *Salmonella* bacteria are destroyed. Scrambled eggs, omelets, and frittatas are properly cooked when no visible liquid egg remains, and any fried eggs you serve should have thickened yolks and whites that are completely set.

Palmar grasp: Serve hard-boiled eggs quartered lengthwise into four vertical wedges, or strips of omelet, fried egg, or quiche measuring ½ inch by 1 inch by 3 inches.

Pincer grasp: Cut quiche, omelets, or hard-boiled, scrambled, or fried eggs into bite-size pieces about 1 square centimeter in size.

Notable Nutrients: Choline and Zinc

Choline plays a crucial role in cell membrane structure, brain development, and brain cell function. Many of the recommended first foods for babies during BLW are top choline sources:

- Beans
- Beef
- Eggs
- Fish
- Soybeans

Zinc is an essential mineral that plays an important role in your baby's immune function as well as overall infant growth and development. One of the best ways to support your baby's immune system is to regularly offer food sources of zinc in the diet. There is no need to overthink it, though. Luckily, many of the recommended iron-rich first foods for babies also contain plenty of zinc. Here are a few examples:

- Beans
- Beef
- Eggs
- Fortified breakfast cereals
- Nuts
- Pork
- Poultry
- Shellfish

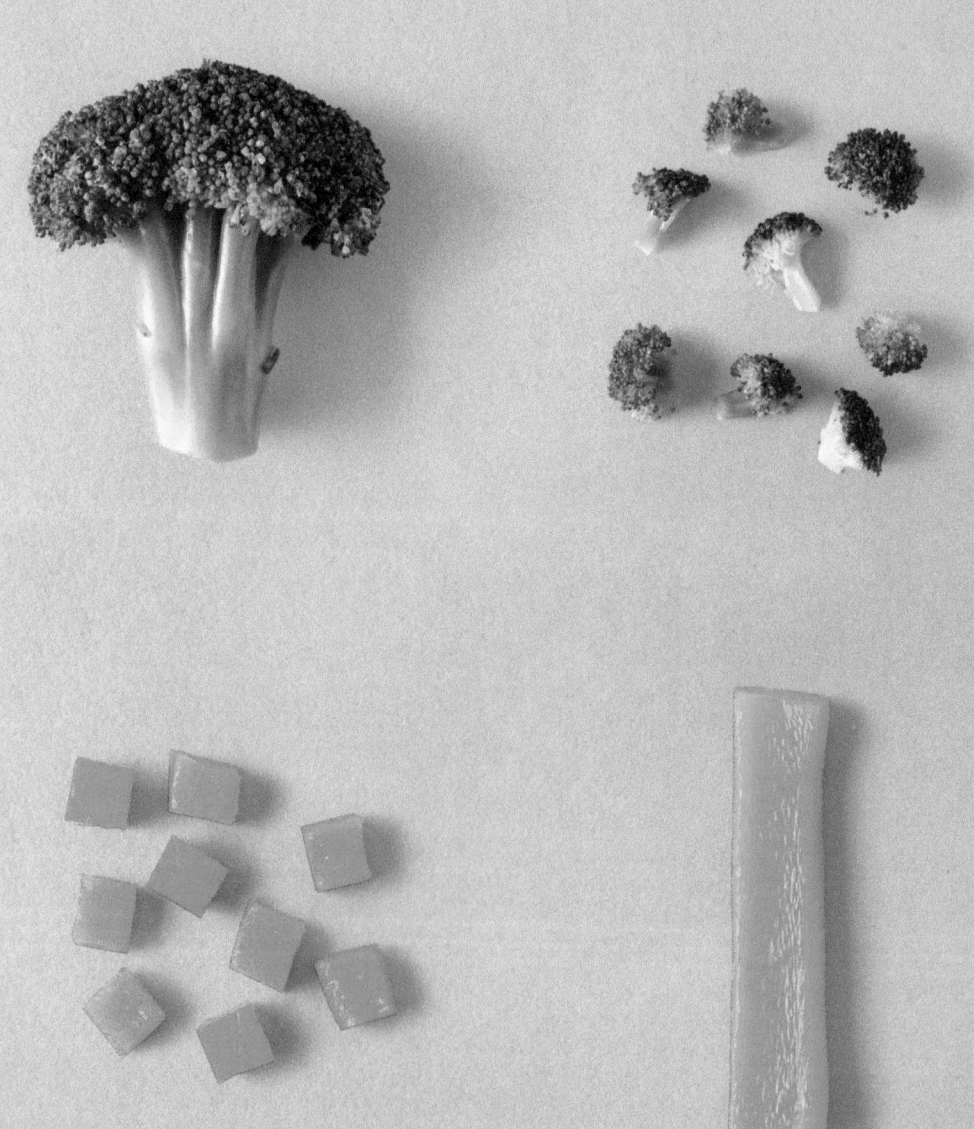

Vegetables and Fruits

Before serving any vegetables and fruits to your baby, be sure to check that they can be easily smashed between your thumb and forefinger. Steam, roast, and sauté veggies until they are tender, and do not be afraid to season them with olive oil, butter, herbs, spices, Parmesan cheese, lemon juice, lemon zest, or bread crumbs. The more flavors you can introduce, the better!

Broccoli

This cruciferous vegetable is an excellent source of vitamin C, which helps improve iron absorption.

Palmar grasp: Offer the tender-cooked whole stem and floret. The stem makes a natural handle so that your baby can grasp it easily and nibble off the top. Once your baby has eaten the floret, take away the stem, which can pose a choking risk.

Pincer grasp: Continue offering the whole stem with the floret or cut it into chickpea-size pieces.

Red Peppers

Red peppers are an excellent source of vitamin C. When they are roasted, their soft texture becomes ideal for babies.

Palmar grasp: Cut into adult pinky-finger-size sticks and roast, or cook them until they can be easily mashed.

Pincer grasp: Cut into chickpea-size, tender-cooked bites.

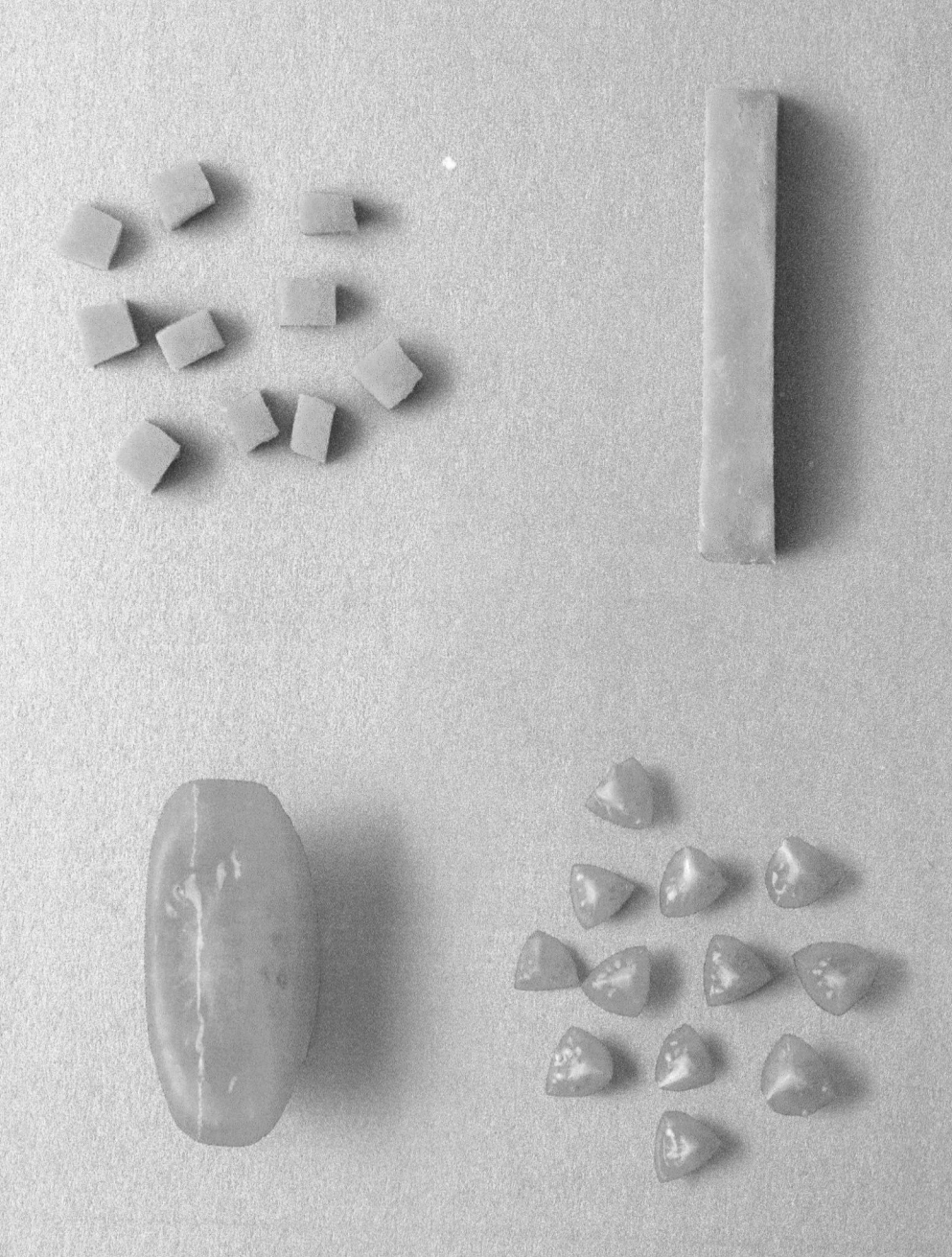

Sweet Potatoes

These starchy, fiber-rich vegetables support digestive health and are highly palatable. Packed with nutrients, they are high in potassium and vitamin A and contain vitamins C and E, folate, copper, iron, and calcium.

Palmar grasp: Peel and cut into adult pinky-finger-size sticks. Cook them until they can be easily mashed. Try using a crinkle cutter to prepare sweet potatoes and other vegetables with similar textures; this creates a shape that makes it easier for babies to grip.

Pincer grasp: Cut into chickpea-size, tender-cooked bites.

Tomatoes

Tomatoes are a good source of vitamin C. When fully ripe, they can be soft enough to serve raw although it is also fine to serve them as a cooked tomato sauce with pasta or as a dip. If you want to serve grape or cherry tomatoes, cut them into quarters.

Palmar grasp: Cut a soft, ripe tomato into wedges that are about $1/2$ inch wide.

Pincer grasp: Continue serving wedges or cut into chickpea-size bites.

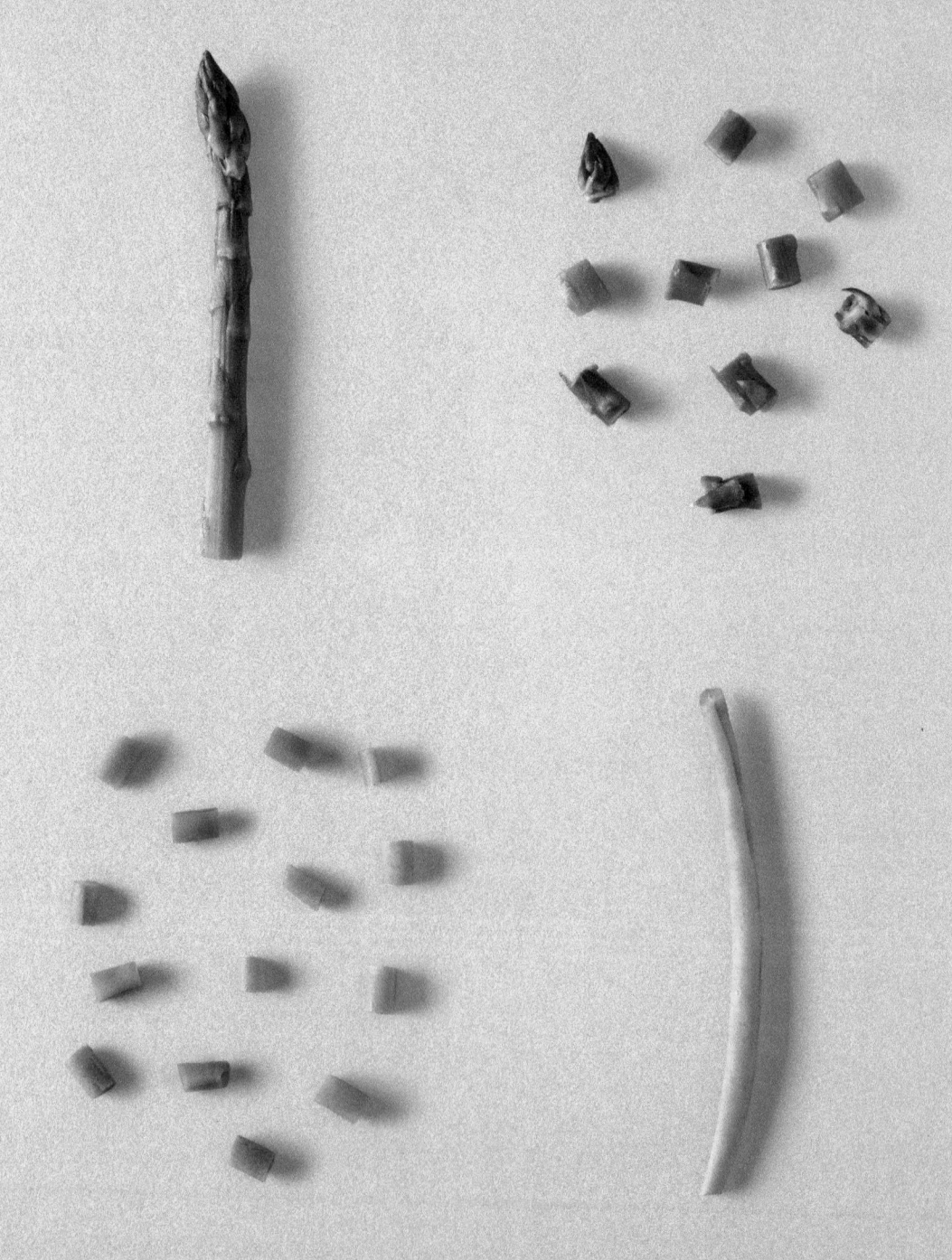

Asparagus

Asparagus offers vitamin C as well as vitamins A, E, and K. Did you know that when asparagus is served without sauce, it is considered proper etiquette to eat it with your fingers no matter how old you are?

Palmar grasp: Offer tender-cooked whole asparagus stalks.

Pincer grasp: Continue offering tender-cooked whole stalks or chickpea-size bites. Oddly enough, all three of my babies had different preferences for bite-size pieces versus whole stalks. Yours likely will, too!

Green Beans

Green beans are naturally sized conveniently for babies and offer a good amount of both vitamin C and iron.

Palmar grasp: Offer tender-cooked, whole trimmed green beans.

Pincer grasp: Continue offering tender-cooked, whole green beans or cut them into bites measuring about ½ inch long.

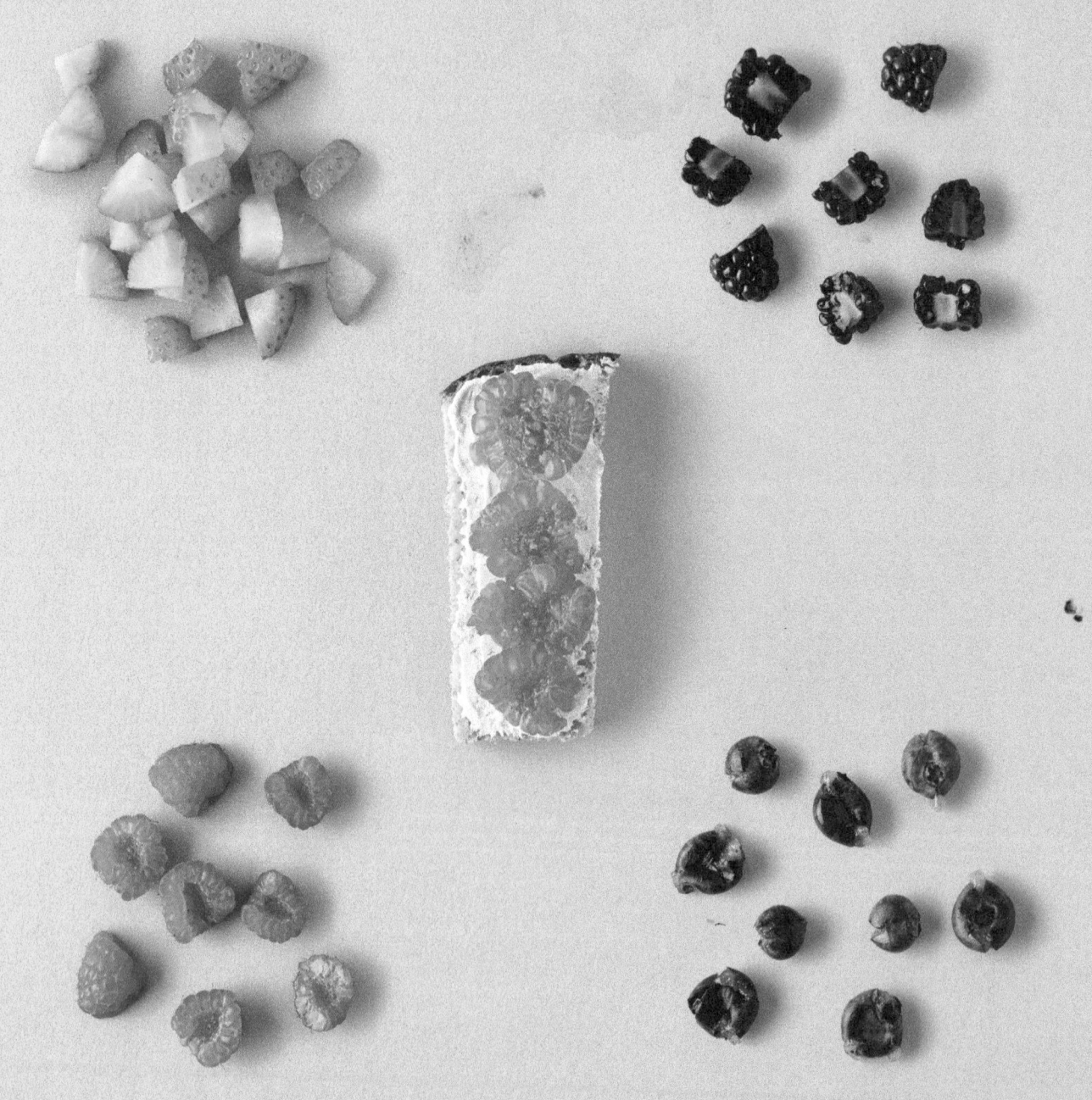

Berries

Strawberries are an excellent source of vitamin C. Frozen, defrosted strawberries are a great texture at this stage, and the cold temperature can be soothing for sore, teething gums. Blueberries, blackberries, and raspberries also offer plenty of vitamin C. Because these are smaller pieces of fruit, they can be difficult for babies who use a palmar grasp.

Palmar grasp: Smash or spread the berries on toast fingers that you have coated with a thin layer of nut butter, soft goat cheese, or cream cheese.

Pincer grasp: Chop soft strawberries into small, chickpea-size bites or offer slices of fresh, soft-ripe, or frozen and defrosted strawberries. Cut ripe raspberries and blueberries in half and ripe blackberries into quarters. Another option that is often easier and faster than cutting is to offer these berries already smashed.

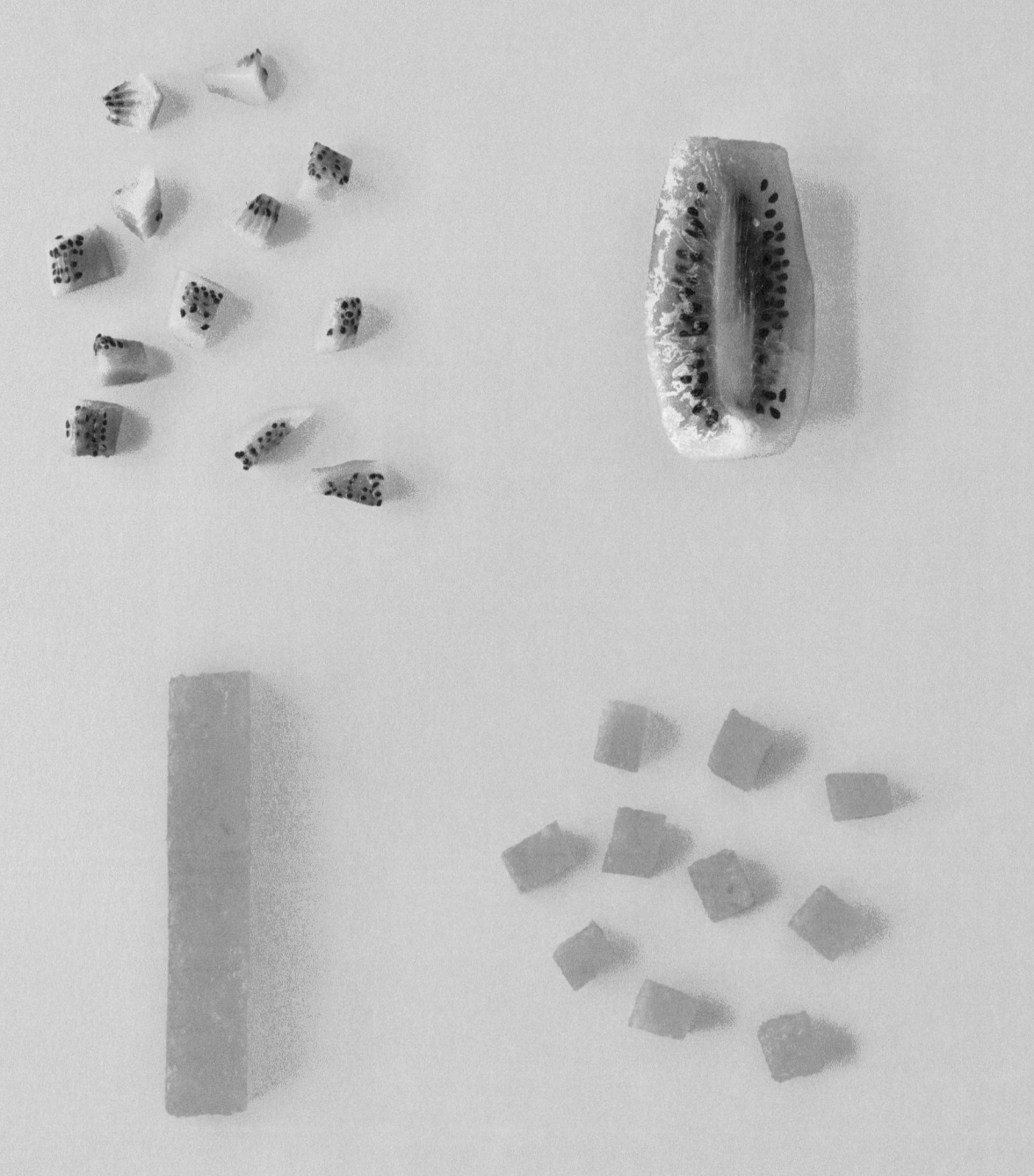

Kiwi

Kiwi fruits are excellent sources of vitamin C. Be sure that any kiwi you serve is very ripe and soft. Remove the hard center core as well as the peel before serving.

Palmar grasp: Offer sliced fingers of fresh, soft-ripe kiwi that are wide enough for your baby to get palms around. If kiwi fingers are too slippery for your baby to pick up, roll them in some sesame seeds, hemp hearts, ground flaxseeds, or a bit of unsweetened, shredded coconut for easier gripping.

Pincer grasp: Continue offering fingers of kiwi or chop soft kiwi into small, chickpea-size bites.

Watermelon

Watermelon is an excellent source of vitamin C. Be sure that it is very ripe and soft, that you have cut it away from the rind, and that you have removed any large seeds before serving.

Palmar grasp: Offer adult pinky-finger-size sticks.

Pincer grasp: Continue offering sticks or chop into small, chickpea-size bites.

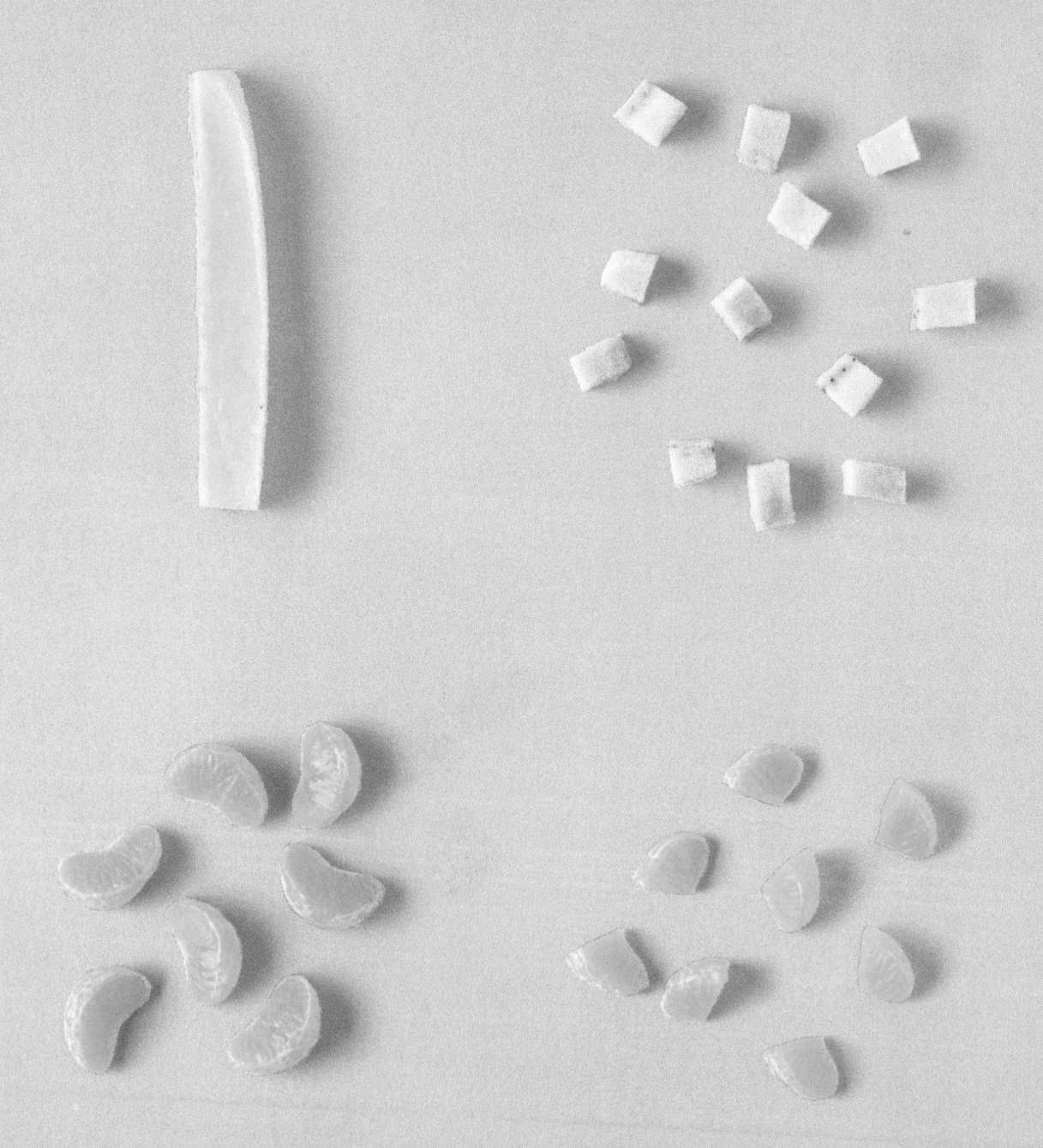

Banana

The texture of very ripe banana is ideal for babies.

Palmar or Pincer grasp: You can offer adult pinky-finger-size strips of ripe banana, or even half of a very ripe banana without the peel, although offering it peeled only half-way down can help give babies a better grip. If you offer it with any part of the peel, be sure to wash the skin before serving. If your baby eats down to the peel, take it away and remove the peel before offering more.

Citrus Fruits

Citrus fruits like oranges are excellent sources of vitamin C, but segments and inner skins can be difficult for babies to negotiate.

Palmar or Pincer grasp: Mandarin oranges canned in water are a good choice for babies who use a pincer grasp. If you serve fresh citrus fruits, take care to remove the peel, seeds, and inner skins, then segment and cut into chickpea-size bites.

Organic Versus Conventional Produce

A common question when parents are starting their babies on solids is whether organically grown foods are healthier for babies than those that are conventionally grown. Whether to buy and serve organic foods is really a personal choice that depends on many factors. When you need to make decisions about which foods to buy and serve to your family, it helps to have some context and know the pertinent facts.

Current research in *Environmental Health* and *Annals of Internal Medicine* shows that the nutrient composition of both organically and conventionally grown foods is comparable and that organic produce does not offer significant nutritional benefits over conventional. This topic, however, continues to be hotly debated. A 2002 study in *Critical Reviews in Food Science and Nutrition* and a 2007 study in the *Journal of Food Science* also show no significant difference in flavor between organically and conventionally grown foods.

The areas where organic and conventionally grown foods tend to differ are price and environmental sustainability. Organic farming practices are healthier for the environment and more supportive of animal welfare, although not exclusively. Organic growing methods tend to enrich the soil rather than leach it of nutrients. These organic growing methods produce less per crop and require more time than conventional growing methods, and this contributes to the higher price of organic foods.

Whether you choose conventional or organic produce, you can reduce your exposure to pesticide residues by thoroughly washing all produce (including organic) before eating and, better yet, by growing your own food in a home garden. If you can afford and want to buy organic, then buy organic. If your resources are limited or you do not want to spend the extra money for organic, know that conventionally grown produce is also a fine choice for you and your family. Bottom line—it is better any day of the week to enjoy a greater variety and volume of conventionally grown than a small or limited amount of organically grown fruits and vegetables.

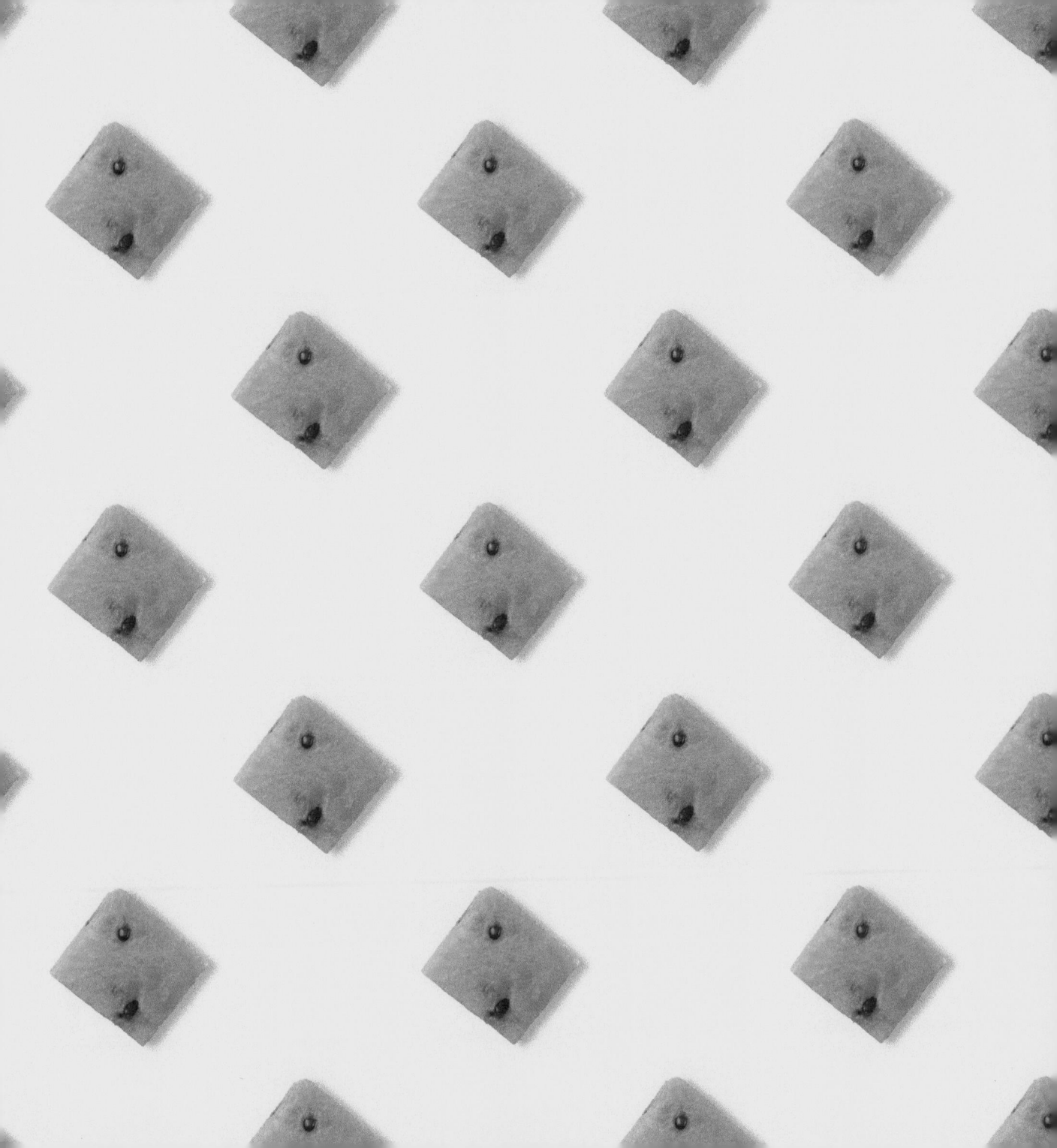

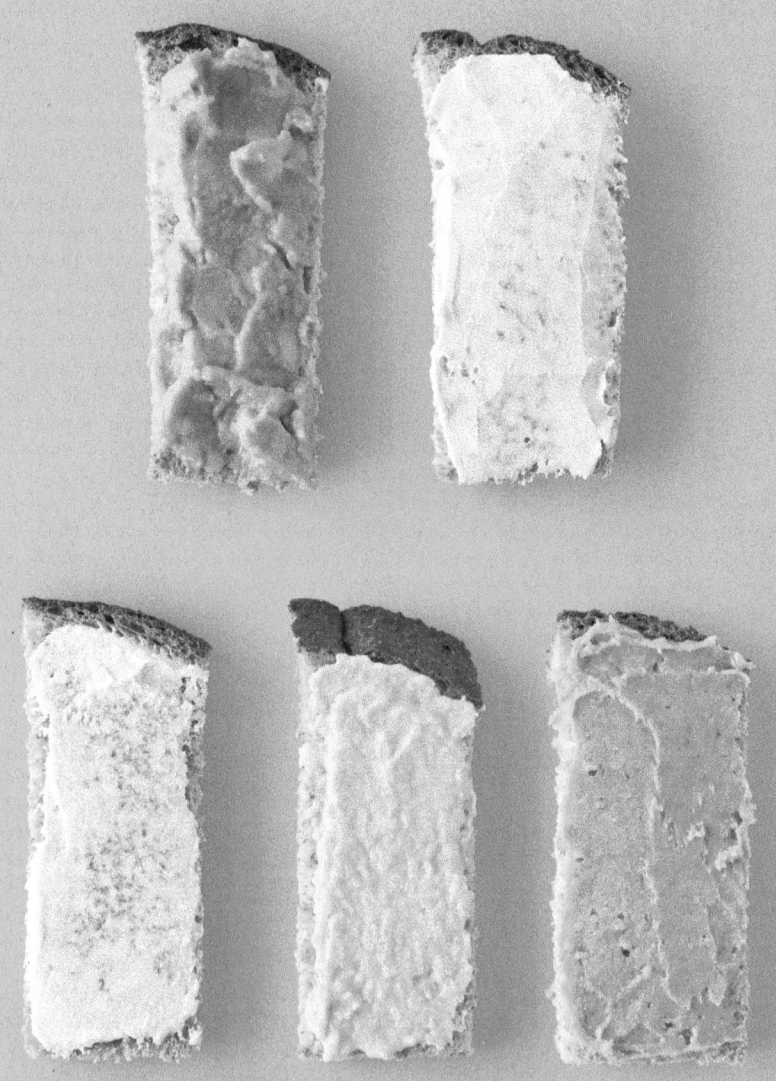

Energy-Rich Foods

Between their newly emerging self-feeding skills and how little they can fit into their small tummies, babies can eat only a small amount of food at a time. Thus, it is important to maximize the nutrients in every bite. The following energy-rich foods are packed with both calories and nutrients to help your baby thrive and grow. In addition to their role as an important part of a balanced meal, many of these foods are also great portable snack options for when you and your baby are on the go.

Toast

Toasted whole-grain bread is a great vehicle for mashed avocado, thinly spread nut butter with smashed berries or bananas, butter, cream cheese, hummus, or bean dip. Many breads tend to be too high in sodium, however, so look for ones with no added salt. (The National Academies of Sciences, Engineering, and Medicine's recommended sodium intake limit for infants 6 to 12 months old is 370 milligrams per day.)

Avoid moist white breads, which can form a gummy ball in the mouth (a choking hazard), as well as overly crusty breads that can be difficult for babies to gum or chew. The key is finding a low-sodium bread that is soft enough for babies to manage but firm enough to grasp. Sprouted-grain, sandwich-type breads that you find in the freezer section of grocery stores often work well. Toast it lightly (not heavily) so that the bread has a bit of give, is not mushy, and does not easily crack off into smaller pieces.

Palmar or Pincer grasp: Cut into fingers measuring 3 inches by 1 inch, add toppings, and offer one finger at a time.

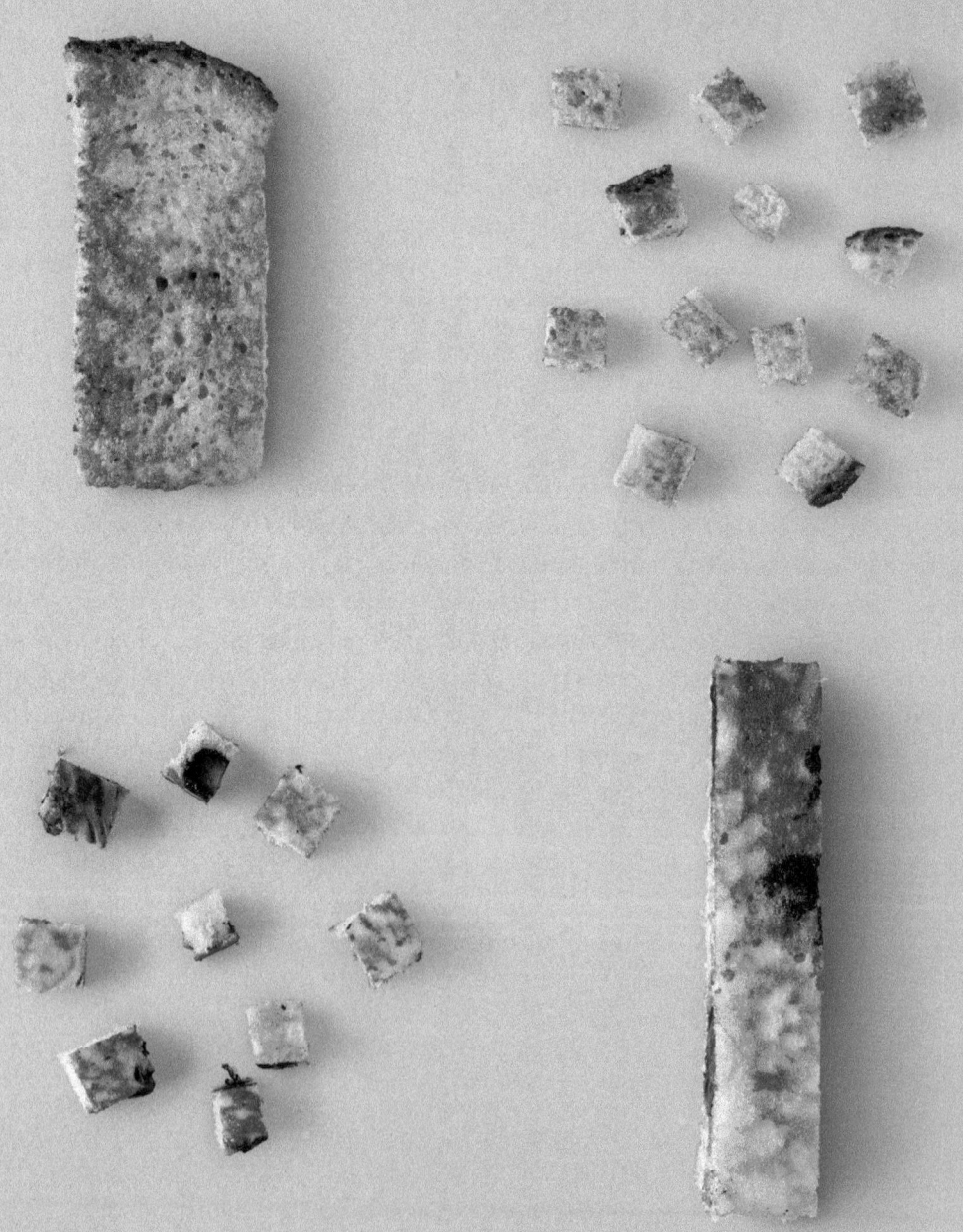

French Toast

A variation on toast fingers, bread soaked in an egg-and-milk mixture and then cooked offers a rich source of many nutrients as well as a great texture and consistency for babies. Do not offer maple syrup at this stage. Smashed berries or other fruits are fine, but added sugars like maple syrup are not recommended for babies under age 1.

Palmar grasp: Cut into fingers measuring 3 inches by 1 inch and offer one finger at a time.

Pincer grasp: Once your baby develops a pincer grasp, you can continue offering toast fingers, or you could chop up the toast into small bites about the width of an adult thumbnail.

Pancakes

Pancakes are an easy way for babies to enjoy many different nutrients, flavors, and new foods. If you have a blender, there is no limit to the potential variations in batter ingredients, including interesting, nutrient-dense combinations like pumpkin with oat, lemon with allspice and hazelnuts, and banana with ricotta cheese. Savory pancakes made with legumes and vegetables are also ideal. If you prefer to use a pancake mix, opt for a whole-grain version so that your baby gets used to the flavor of whole grains rather than those that are more refined. Skip the maple syrup and instead serve the pancakes with mashed fruit, or add chopped fruit directly into the pancake batter before cooking.

Palmar grasp: Cut into fingers measuring 3 inches by 1 inch and offer one finger at a time.

Pincer grasp: Continue offering pancake fingers or cut into smaller pieces about the size of a chickpea.

Fresh Versus Frozen Versus Canned

You may have questions about whether it is healthier to serve fresh, frozen, or canned produce. In general, the more fruits and vegetables in your family's diet, the better!

Buying a blend of fresh, frozen, and canned is more affordable and convenient, which can make it easier to serve fruits and vegetables more frequently. Fresh produce is generally best, but it perishes faster and certain types are available only seasonally. Frozen produce is a fantastic option because it lasts longer in the freezer, and it is usually picked at peak ripeness and flash-frozen immediately, which helps retain maximum nutrient content and extend storage time.

Canned produce ranges from nutrient-dense to heavily processed, but it is often more widely available and more affordable. You can avoid added sugars by choosing fruits that are canned in water or fruit juice rather than syrup. Avoid excess sodium by choosing canned vegetables with package claims such as "no salt added" or "reduced sodium."

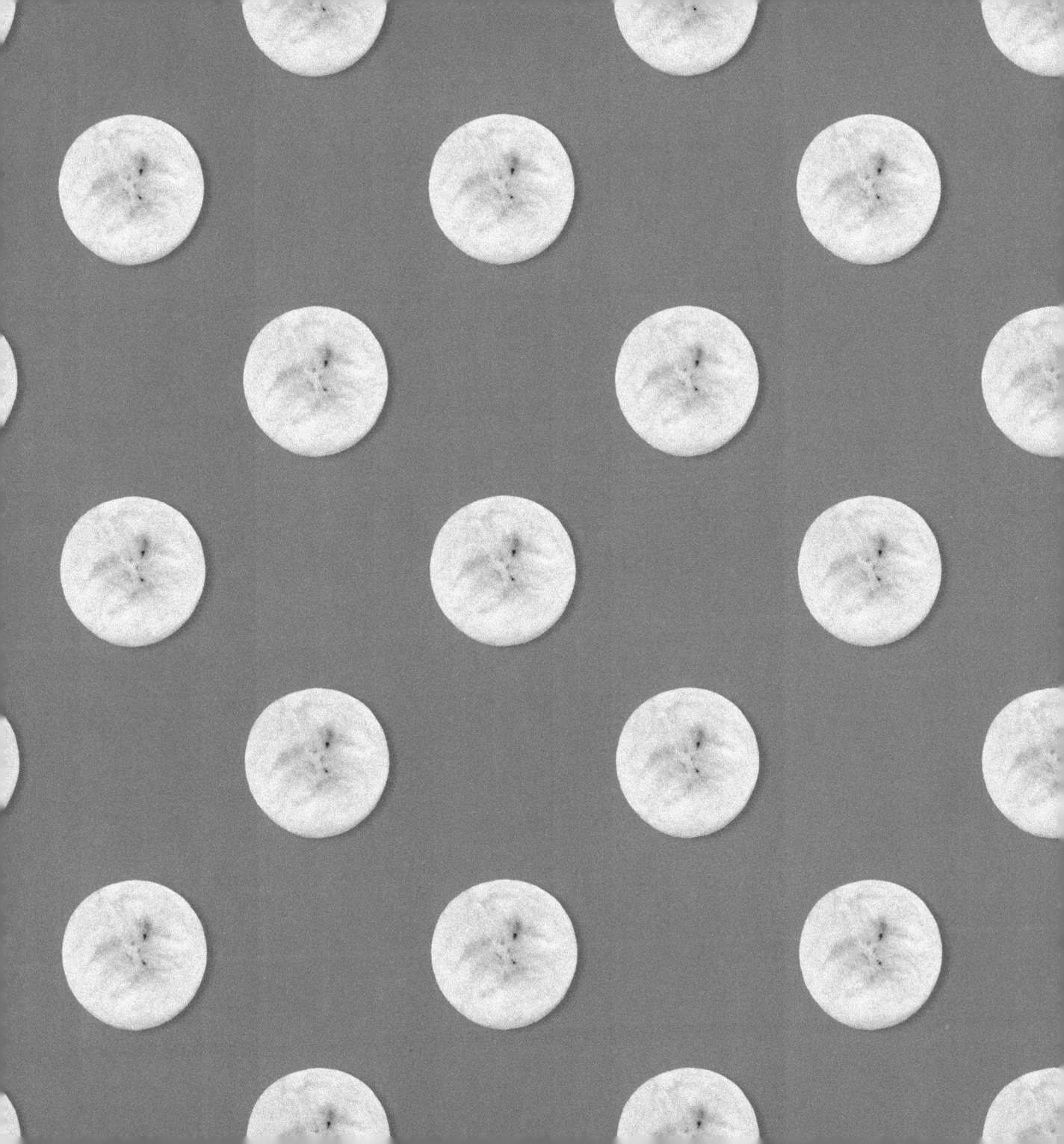

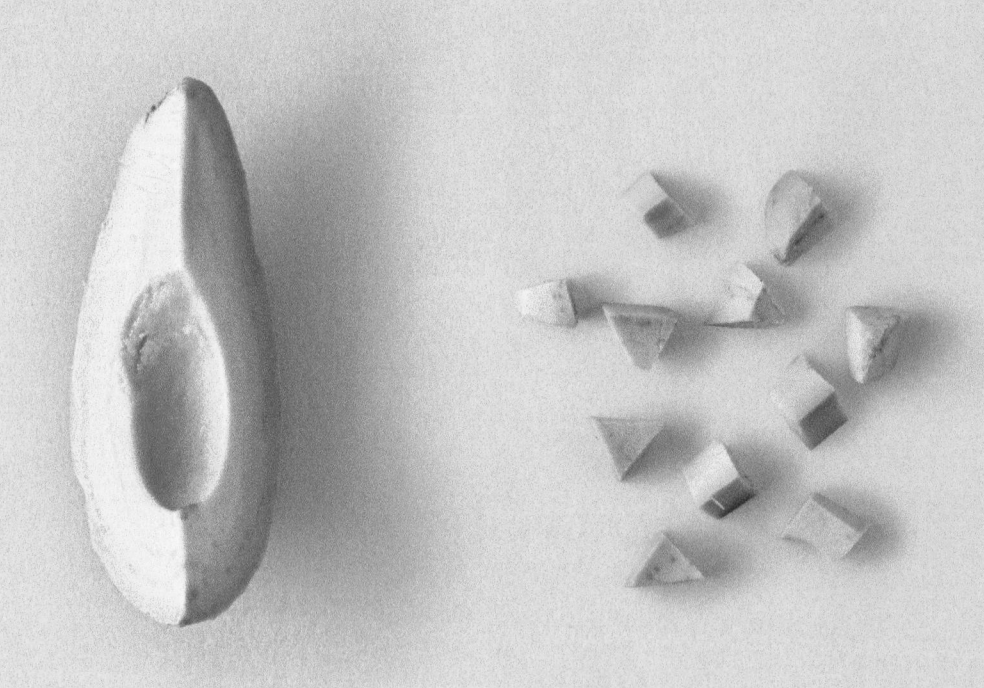

Avocado

Although technically a fruit, avocado makes it onto the list of energy-rich foods because it is high in both calories and healthy fats. Ripe avocado is easily mashed, soft, tasty, and nutrient-dense, making it one of the best first foods for babies.

Palmar grasp: Offer peeled, sliced wedges of fresh, soft-ripe avocado. If it is too slippery for your baby to grasp, roll it in some unsweetened, shredded coconut, hemp hearts, or ground flaxseeds for easier gripping.

Pincer grasp: Chop ripe avocado into small, chickpea-size bites.

Notable Nutrient: Probiotics

Probiotics are a hot topic and an area of emerging research these days. You have probably heard of them—the friendly bacteria that live in the gut, help with digestion, and may contribute to overall human health in many ways. Probiotics can pass from mother to baby in breast milk and are found in fermented foods such as yogurt, kimchi, sauerkraut, kefir, and miso.

There is not a lot of research on probiotics and infants. In fact, there is still a lot we do not know about probiotics in general. Most of the available research indicates that they are safe for healthy infants, and a 2013 study in *BMC Pediatrics* suggests that probiotics may benefit infants with colic and certain gastrointestinal conditions. You may have read that probiotics have the potential to help with food allergies; although there is some promising research in this area, trials so far have shown only mixed or unclear effects of the ability of probiotics to prevent food and environmental allergies as well as asthma.

In any case, no major medical organizations have endorsed the use of probiotic supplements in infants, and there is currently no official recommended dose for infants, so be sure to check with your pediatrician or registered dietitian before deciding to start your baby on any type of probiotic supplement. Anyone with a weakened immune system or health issue can have an adverse reaction to probiotics, which come in many different strains and formulas. Government regulation of probiotics is complicated in that it depends on whether the intended use of the probiotic product is that of a supplement, food ingredient, or drug. An option that works well for many families is integrating more probiotic-containing foods into the entire family's diet, so that everyone benefits. Fermented foods like yogurt, kimchi, sauerkraut, kefir, and miso offer a range of healthy nutrients and a variety of friendly bacteria.

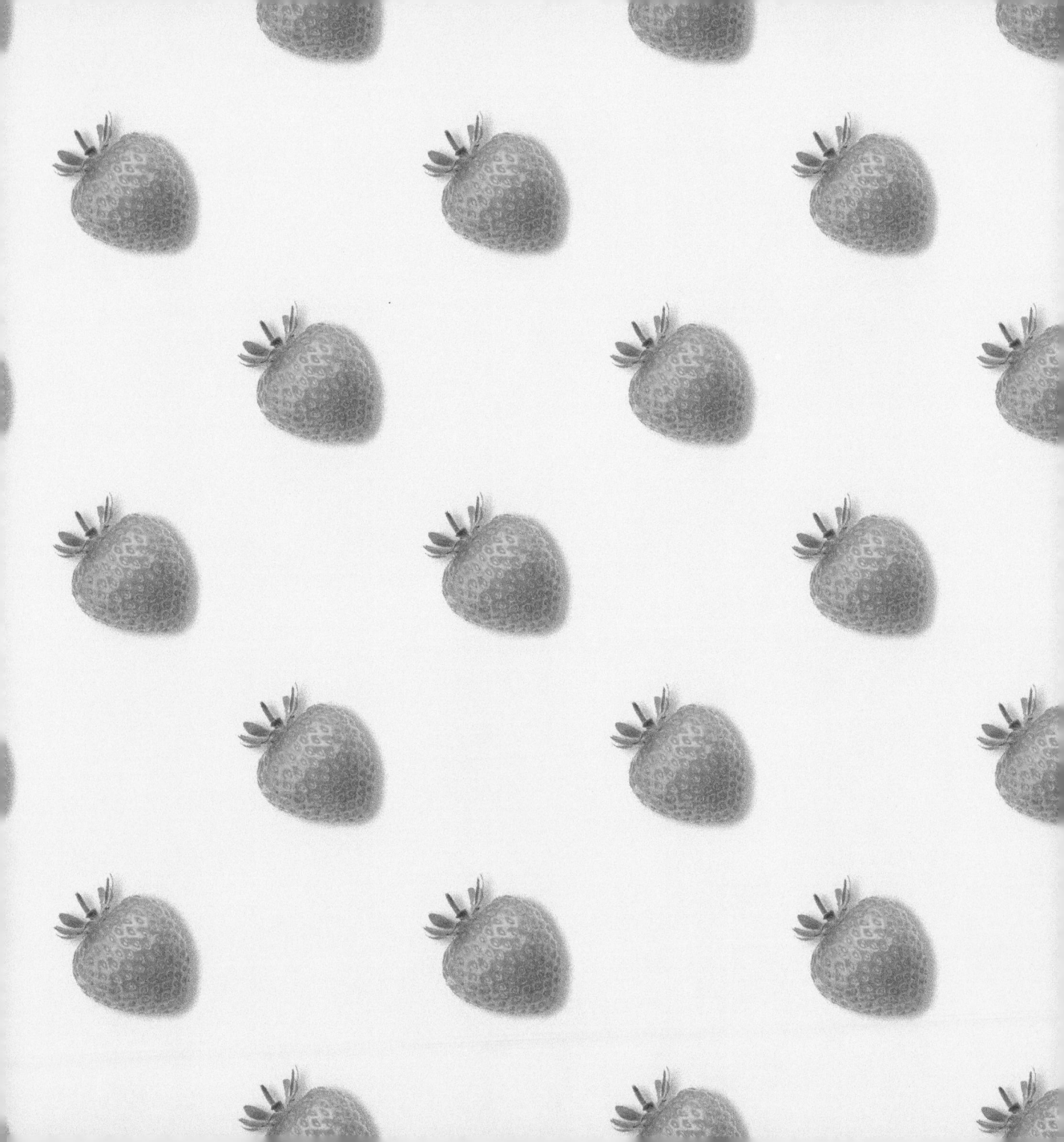

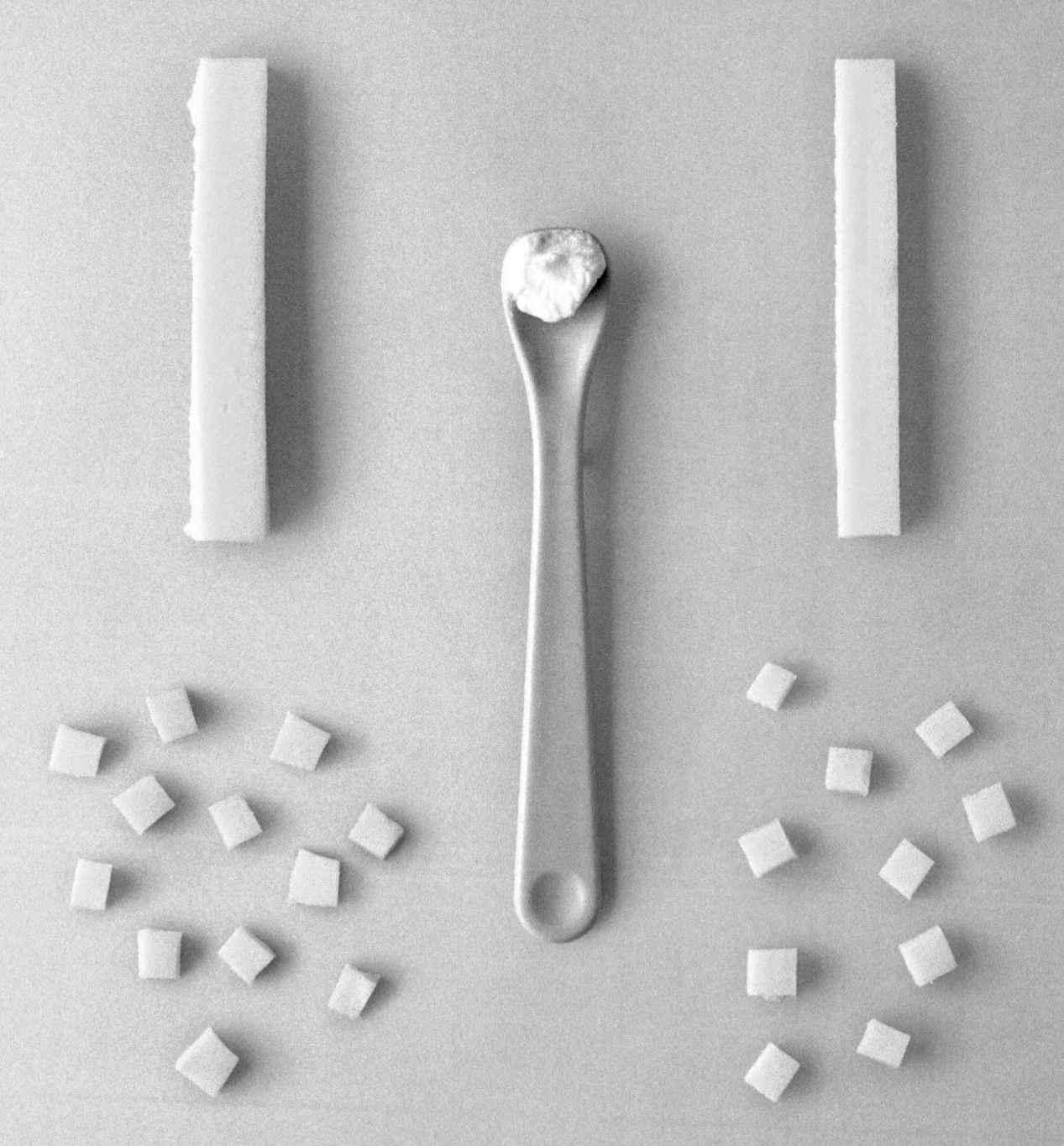

Full-Fat Cheese

Cheese offers plenty of calories, fat, calcium, and other nutrients that promote health in babies, but many types contain 200 milligrams or more of sodium per ounce, which is not ideal for infant kidneys. Check food labels before you buy and choose cheeses that contain around 50 milligrams of sodium or less; some soft cheeses like full-fat ricotta, fresh mozzarella, mascarpone, quark, goat cheese, and crème fraîche tend to be lower in sodium than hard cheeses (although Swiss may be a good choice among the latter). Also, check the labels to make sure that the cheeses are pasteurized, as unpasteurized cheese carries a risk of foodborne illness.

Palmar grasp: Spread soft cheeses on toast fingers, cut Swiss or fresh mozzarella into strips the size of an adult pinky finger, or offer creamy soft cheeses like ricotta and crème fraîche on a preloaded spoon.

Pincer grasp: In addition to the above, you can also cut Swiss or fresh mozzarella cheeses into chickpea-size pieces.

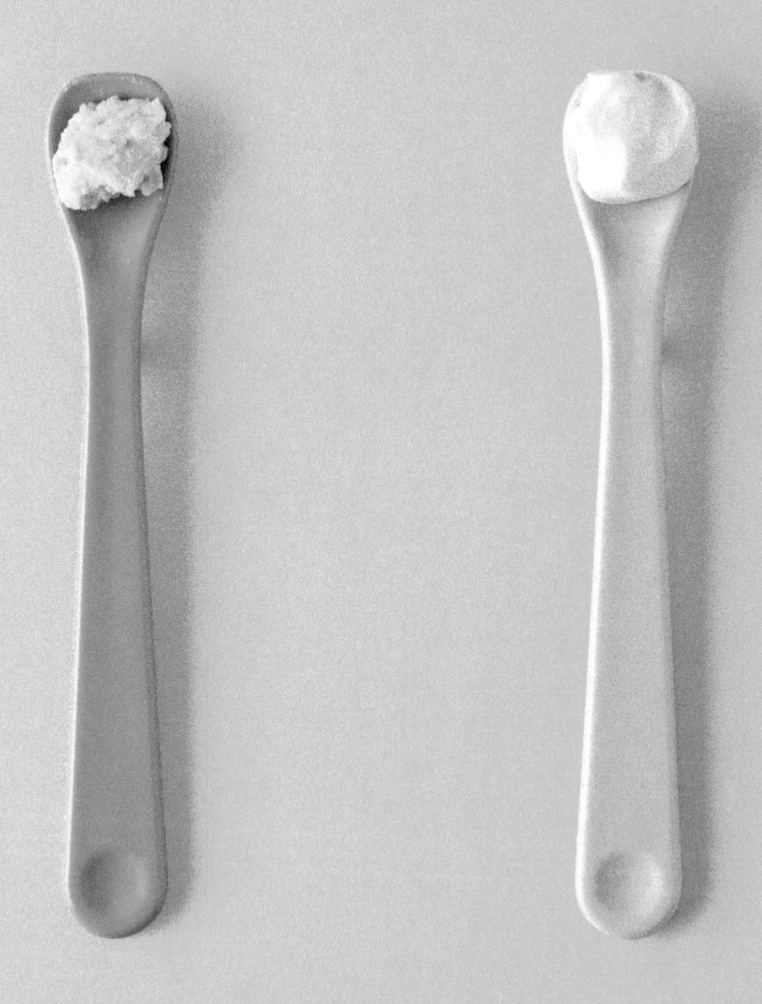

Oatmeal

Oats are one of my favorite grains because they are rich in fiber, contain protein and fat, and are high in many vitamins and minerals, including iron and zinc. You can increase the nutrients and calories in oatmeal for your baby by cooking it in whole cow's milk, soymilk, or pea milk and adding a little butter. Oatmeal is a great vehicle for many other foods as well; consider swirling in a teaspoon of nut butter, hemp hearts, or chopped fruits for an added nutrient boost.

Palmar grasp: Serve thick oatmeal on a preloaded spoon. You can also make a baked oatmeal casserole and cut it into pieces the size of an adult pinky finger.

Pincer grasp: Serve thick oatmeal on a preloaded spoon or serve chickpea-size bites of oatmeal casserole.

Plain, Full-Fat Greek Yogurt

A source of many important nutrients, yogurt also provides probiotics—the "good bacteria" that support gut health, immunity, and digestion. Choose unsweetened plain versions with a label that says "live or active cultures" and serve them on a preloaded spoon. Your baby will soon be able to load the spoon alone. The thicker texture of Greek yogurt makes it easier to keep on the spoon, but do not be surprised if your baby takes a shortcut and ends up scooping handfuls instead.

What's the Deal with Baby Cereals?

For decades, baby rice cereal has been a very common first food for babies who are spoon-fed conventionally. The rationale behind starting 3- to 4-month-old babies on rice cereal was that this bland carbohydrate could be easily spoon-fed, accepted, and digested and therefore was more effective at helping babies gain weight and grow. However, infant rice cereal is actually nutrient-poor, filling, and not easily digestible for babies under 6 months—not an ideal combination, because the cereal often ends up replacing significantly more nourishing options in the baby's diet, such as breast milk or formula.

Another common misconception about baby cereal is that starting babies early on solids like rice cereal will help them begin sleeping through the night. The reality is that night waking in babies happens for all sorts of reasons, and there is no evidence that the early introduction of solids solves the issue.

Once a baby is about 6 months of age and showing true signs of readiness for solid foods, rice and other grain-based baby cereals are fine as long as they are offered as a part of a varied, balanced diet and fed responsively on a preloaded spoon. Iron-fortified baby cereals are also a convenient way during BLW to boost iron intake and thicken puréed textures that won't otherwise stay on a spoon while a baby is self-feeding.

Furthermore, for babies who are at a high risk for food allergies and whose doctors recommend early introduction of certain allergens, these cereals can be helpful because they offer a texture that a younger baby can manage and into which allergens can be mixed. That being said, it is not necessary or advised to offer rice or grain-based baby cereals as a first food. Minimally processed finger foods offer a wider range of both nutritional and experiential benefits, such as new flavors, textures, colors, and aromas, all of which help babies expand their palates and broaden their nutrient intake.

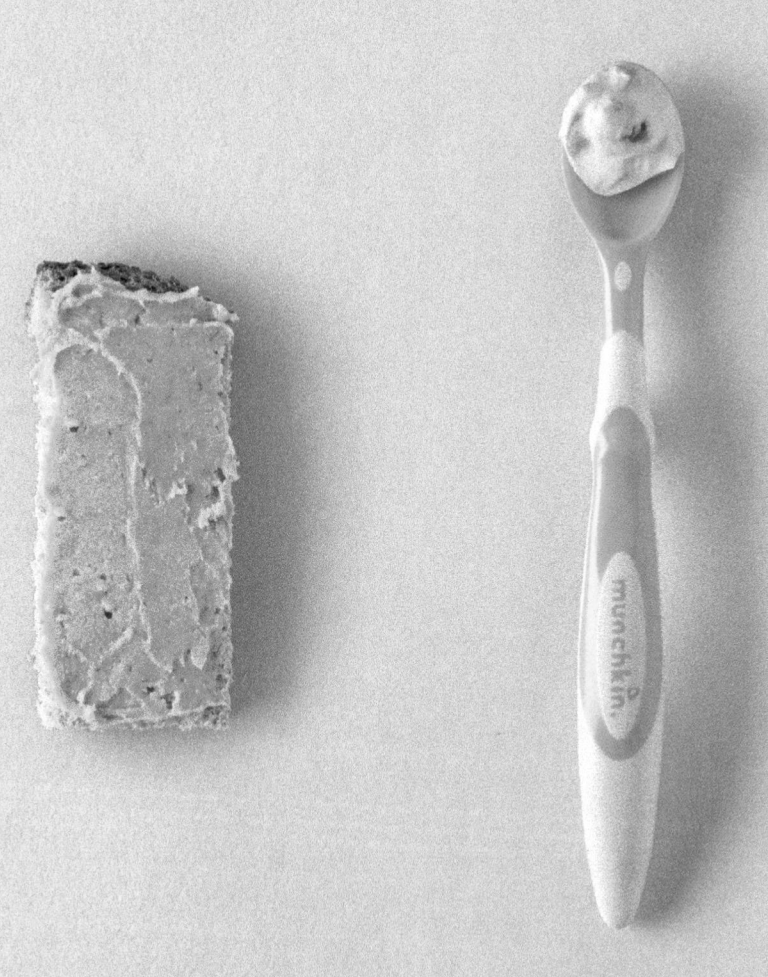

Nuts

Nuts are high in calories and bursting with vitamins, minerals, and antioxidants. They are also a great source of healthy fats, which are crucial for brain development. Although both whole nuts and chunks or spoonfuls of nut butters are choking hazards, there are many safe ways to serve nuts to babies:

- Swirl a teaspoon of nut butter into yogurt or oatmeal.
- Spread a thin layer of nut butter on toast or pancake fingers.
- Blend nut butters into smoothies, pancake batters, muffins, and quick breads.
- Roll meats or vegetables in finely ground almond or hazelnut flours before cooking.

CHAPTER FIVE

FOODS TO AVOID IN YOUR BABY'S FIRST YEAR

Although your baby can eat a wide range of foods during the first year of life, some foods should be avoided for safety reasons.

Here is a list of foods to be conscious of, as well as why they are important not to introduce before your baby's first birthday:

- **Honey** (even in baked or cooked items)

  - Honey can be tainted with a toxin called *Clostridium botulinum* that can cause infant botulism and is dangerous for babies under 1 year of age.
  - As babies grow, their digestive systems mature and can better handle the bacteria before it causes harm.

- **Cow's milk**

  - Cow's milk can inhibit iron absorption.
  - It can also end up replacing breast milk or formula in a baby's diet, which is not advised.
  - Do not worry about offering baked goods, oatmeal, or other recipes made with cow's milk, but avoid offering cow's milk as a beverage until your baby is 12 months old or older.
  - Other dairy foods made with cow's milk, such as yogurt and cottage cheese, are fine.

- **Soft cheeses made with unpasteurized milk (such as goat and feta) and deli meats**

  - These foods can contain a germ called *Listeria monocytogenes.*
  - *Listeria monocytogenes* grows in refrigerator-like temperatures and can lead to an infection called listeria.
  - Avoid offering these foods until your baby is at least 12 months old.

The following foods are choking hazards and should be avoided for **at least** the first year of life:

- Hard candies
- Whole grapes and cherry or grape tomatoes (should be quartered before serving)
- Hard, round nuts (including hazelnuts, macadamia nuts, almonds, pecans, cashews, and Brazil nuts)
- Fruits with stones such as peaches, plums, nectarines, apricots, and cherries (remove the pit and cut into appropriate sizes before serving)
- Popcorn
- Any hard, coin-shaped foods (hot dogs, sausages, carrot rounds)
- Raw leafy greens (such as raw spinach, kale, bok choy, collard greens, Swiss chard)
- Moist white bread
- Overly dry or crusty bread (especially thickly cut), with or without spread
- Nut and seed butters that are thickly spread or in spoonfuls (thin layers are fine)
- Marshmallows
- Dried fruits: Larger raisins and other roundish dried fruits like apricots, prunes, figs, dates, and peaches pose a choking risk, but they are also energy-rich and many contain significant amounts of iron. Note: You can serve these fruits to babies who have developed a pincer grasp by first soaking them in hot water for about 5 minutes and then chopping them into chickpea-size bites.
- Raw apples (whole or sliced) and any underripe hard fruits or vegetables with tough skins are choking hazards. Instead, serve them peeled and grated or tender-cooked.

Nutrients to Limit

Nutrients to limit when you prepare food for your baby include added salt and added sugars. Your baby's kidneys are not able to process large amounts of sodium. You can avoid having too much sodium in your baby's diet by avoiding processed foods, steering clear of the saltshaker, and even setting aside a portion of a recipe for your baby before you add salt.

Added sugars, which include refined white sugar, agave syrup, maple syrup, and honey, are nutrient-poor and should not be offered to babies under the age of 1. Babies do have a natural affinity for sweet-tasting foods, but at this stage, their infant palates are perhaps the most open they will ever be to nonsweet flavors like bitter, sour, and savory. It is okay to offer naturally sweet foods like fruits, which also offer a wide range of healthy nutrients, but skip the added sugars so that your baby can learn to appreciate many other flavors as well.

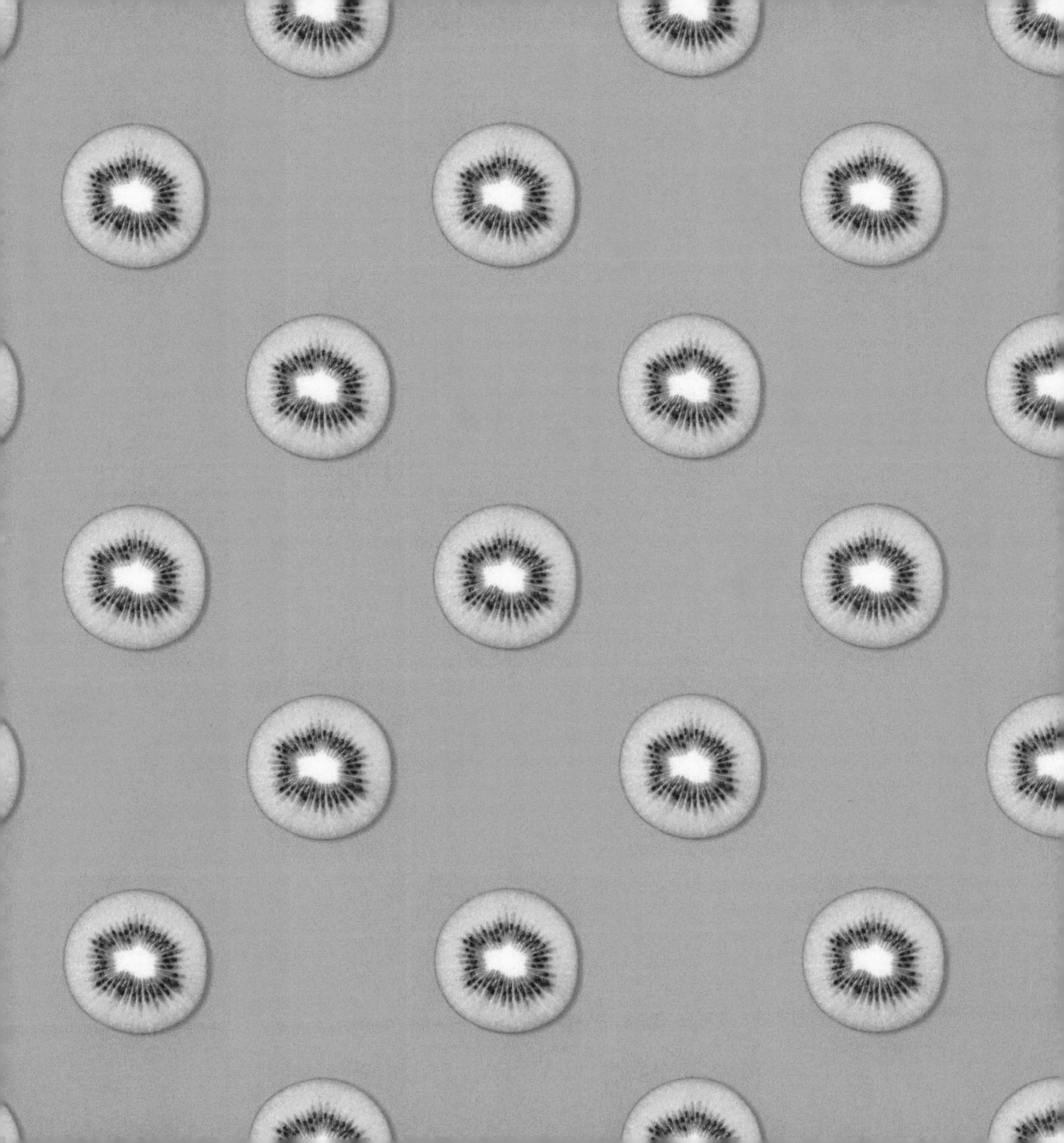

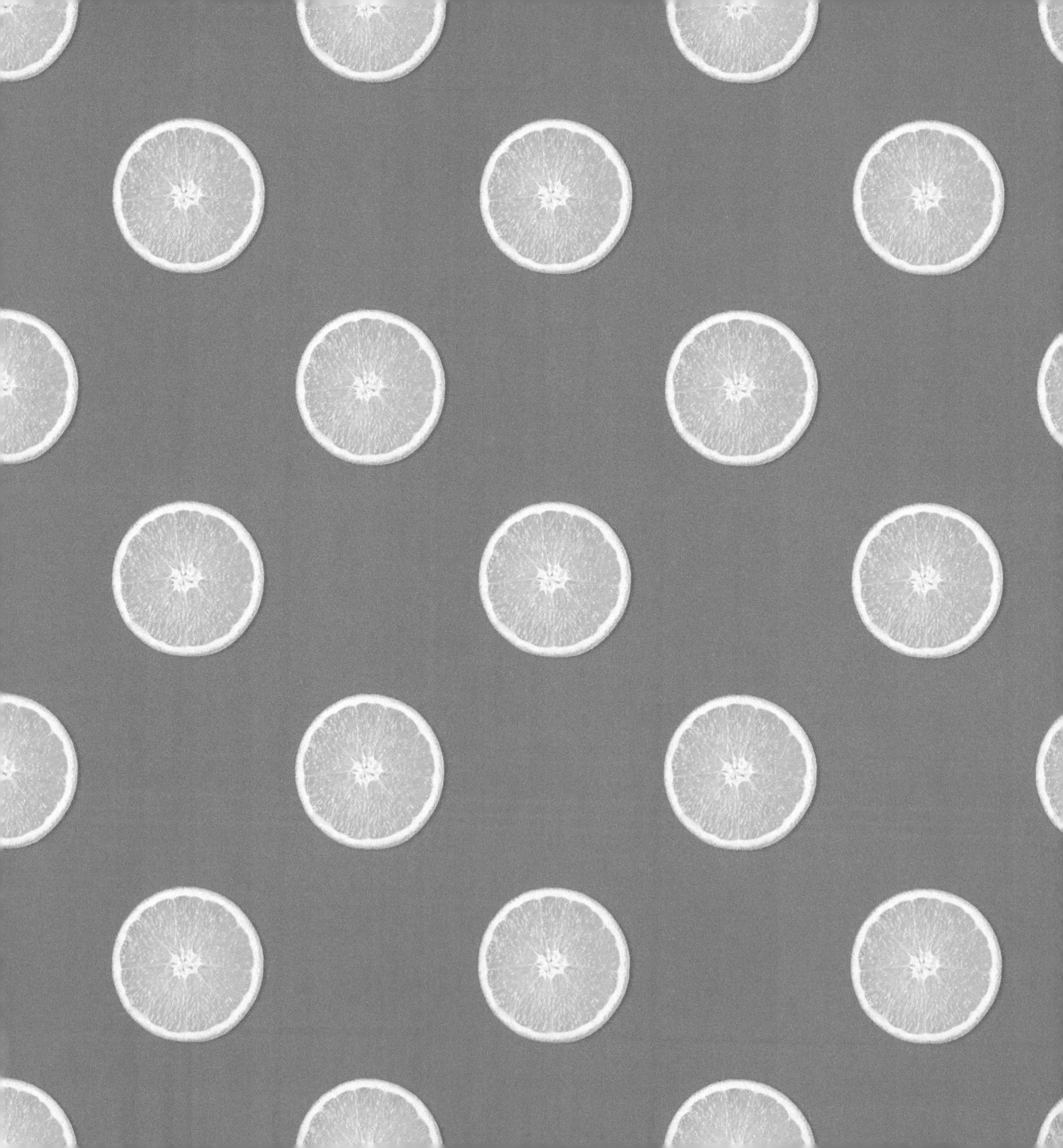

PART THREE

UNDERSTANDING FOOD ALLERGIES & SENSITIVITIES

One of the most frequently asked questions in the world of infant feeding is how to navigate potential food allergies. We know now that in addition to genes and environment, early infant nutrition affects how food allergies develop. As a result, recommendations have changed in response to the latest research, so it is important to stay current.

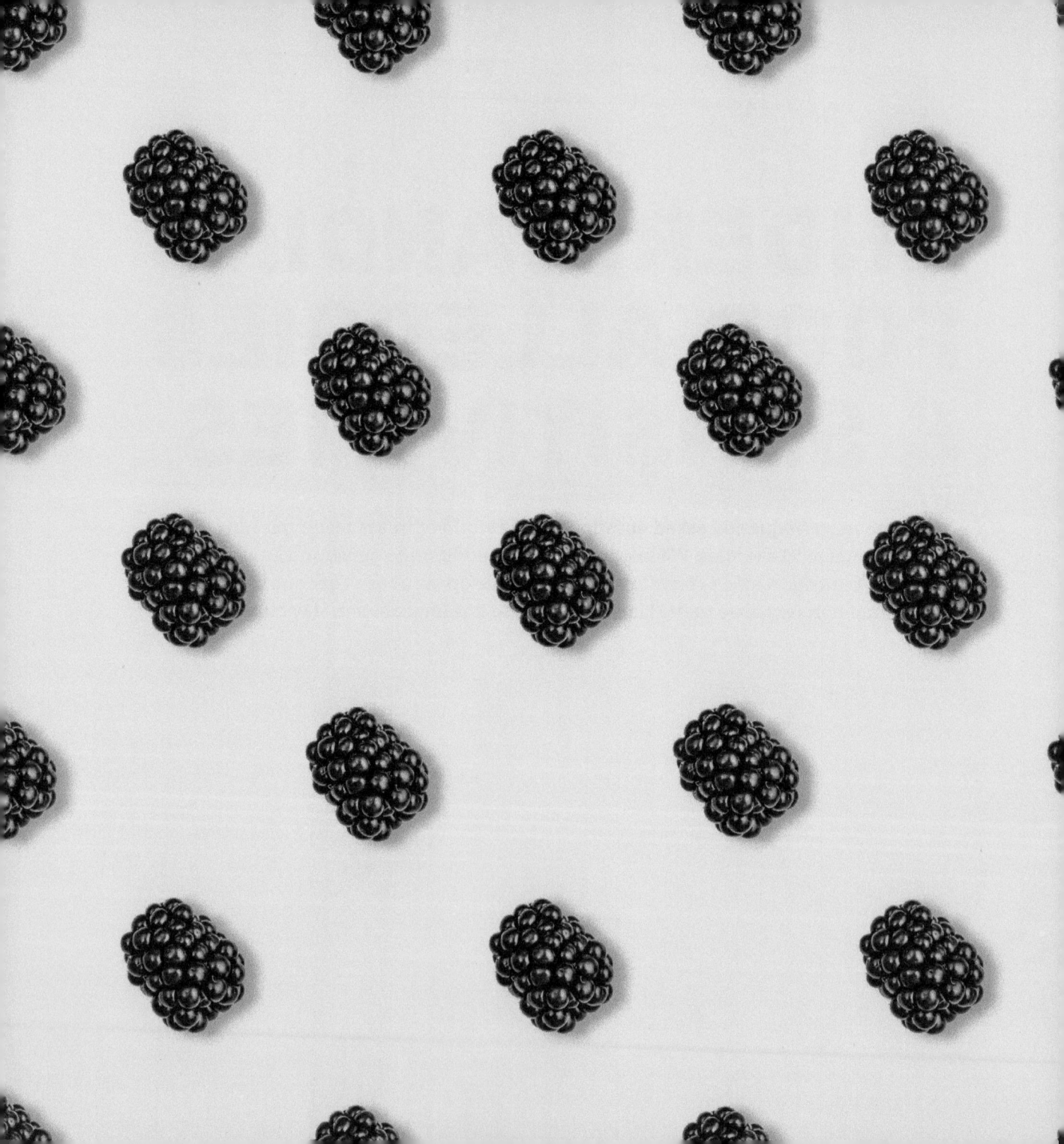

CHAPTER SIX

WHY DO FOOD ALLERGIES OCCUR?

A food allergy occurs when the body's immune system mistakenly identifies part of a food (usually a protein) as a threat and responds with an adverse reaction. Any organ system can be affected during a food allergy reaction, including the skin, cardiovascular system, gastrointestinal tract, and respiratory system. Some reactions can be life-threatening.

In a typical food allergy reaction, immunoglobulin E (IgE) antibodies trigger the release of chemicals in the body such as histamine, which cause the symptoms associated with allergies. These reactions usually happen within minutes of ingestion but they can also take up to 2 hours. IgE-mediated reactions can be life-threatening; however, non-IgE reactions involve other parts of the immune system, typically cause delayed reactions within a few hours of ingesting the food, and are not life-threatening.

According to a 2018 study in *Pediatrics*, 8 percent of children have a convincing food allergy, and of that 8 percent, 42 percent have reported a severe reaction and 40 percent are allergic to multiple foods. According to the National Institute of Allergy and Infectious Disease, by age 5, most kids outgrow allergies to milk, egg, soy, and wheat and a smaller percentage outgrow peanut and tree nut allergies. Outgrowing an allergy can happen as late as adolescence, but some allergies are lifelong. Food allergies have no known cure, although experimental immunotherapies that are currently undergoing clinical trials may reduce symptoms in some people.

The Eight Most Common Allergenic Foods

Over 170 foods are known to cause food allergies. Reactions are unpredictable and sensitivities vary. Symptoms can range from mild (hives) to severe (anaphylaxis), and tiny amounts can cause reactions depending on an individual's sensitivity.

According to Food Allergy Research and Education (FARE), the following eight allergens are responsible for nearly 90 percent of all food allergies in the United States (and sesame allergies are on the rise as well):

- Cow's milk
- Eggs
- Fish
- Peanuts
- Shellfish
- Soy
- Tree nuts
- Wheat

In the United States, labels for processed foods must fully disclose if these foods are intentionally included; however, precautionary labeling (such as "manufactured in a facility with") is voluntary and unregulated.

When to Think About Allergies

As you begin BLW, it is important to be aware of the eight most common allergenic foods and follow the most current recommendations on introducing them. Contrary to past guidelines—which recommended avoidance—early introduction is now believed to be one of the best methods of prevention. According to an April 2019 clinical report from the American Academy of Pediatrics, delaying the introduction of allergenic foods beyond 4 to 6 months of age does not appear to prevent or delay food allergies. Most notably, a large randomized clinical trial called Learning Early About Peanut Allergy (LEAP) found that early introduction and subsequent regular intake of peanuts reduce the risk of developing peanut allergy in high-risk infants by 81 percent.

This finding is hugely significant, given statistics reported in a study funded by FARE showing that, between 1997 and 2008, the prevalence of peanut or tree nut allergies in the United States seems to have tripled in children. In 2016, the National Institute of Allergy and Infectious Diseases issued new guidelines on when to introduce an infant-safe form of peanuts, which depends on whether your baby is at risk for food allergies.

Babies have different levels of risk for food allergies, so if you are concerned, be sure to talk with your pediatrician about it during the first 4 months of your baby's life, well before you begin offering your baby solid foods.

How Do I Know If My Baby Is Allergic?

Food allergies can be a complex and confusing topic. The Centers for Disease Control and Prevention report that there has been a 50 percent increase in food allergies in children since the late 1990s, and although there are theories as to why, research has yet to identify the cause of the increase.

Anyone of any age, race, ethnicity, or background can develop a food allergy. Having a family history of asthma, eczema, food allergies, and seasonal or environmental allergies increases the risk, but the strongest risk factors for developing childhood food allergies are eczema in infancy and its level of severity. If your baby has or has had eczema, your pediatrician can tell you whether it is mild, moderate, or severe and guide your next steps toward introducing the top allergenic foods. But be sure to have this discussion early because the research shows that the infants who benefit most from early introduction to allergens are those with known risk factors.

If you have checked with your doctor and your baby is not at risk for food allergies (most babies are not), begin to offer the top eight allergenic foods (page 103) starting at about 6 months of age. Offer them one at a time and not as a part of a mixed dish. Wait about a day or so in between each new allergenic food introduction.

Whether your baby is at risk for food allergies or not, it is always a good idea to familiarize yourself with the signs and symptoms of allergic reactions so that you can respond appropriately should a reaction occur.

Identifying Allergic Reactions

Allergic reactions can range from mild to severe and tend to appear within minutes of consuming the food. Some symptoms, however, can appear several hours later. Common symptoms may appear alone or in combination:

Mild-Moderate Symptoms

- A few hives (or red, warm, raised welts) or itchiness around the mouth or face
- Nausea and vomiting
- Diarrhea
- Stomach pain
- Widespread hives or welts on the body
- Repetitive coughing

Severe Symptoms (may indicate signs of anaphylaxis)

- Swelling of the lips, tongue, and throat that blocks breathing
- Difficulty swallowing or breathing
- Drop in blood pressure
- Sudden tiredness, lethargy, weakness, and confusion
- Loss of consciousness

If you notice any mild or moderate symptoms, contact your pediatrician, who may refer you to an allergist for further evaluation and testing.

If you see any signs of a severe allergic reaction or anaphylaxis, call 911 and seek medical attention immediately. Epinephrine is the only medicine that can stop anaphylaxis and must be administered quickly. **Diphenhydramine (such as Benadryl) will not treat anaphylaxis.**

Although severe reactions are uncommon in infants, they can occur. In 2017, the US Food and Drug Administration approved the first epinephrine auto-injector (EpiPen®) for infants weighing between 16.5 and 33 pounds. If your baby's doctor identifies your baby as being at high risk of anaphylaxis, an EpiPen may be prescribed to ease symptoms in the event of an emergency. Working closely with your pediatrician and board-certified allergist will help you create the right emergency-action plan for your baby.

Food Protein-Induced Enterocolitis Syndrome (FPIES) is a severe, non-IgE–mediated condition based in the gastrointestinal tract; it is sometimes referred to as "delayed food allergy." FPIES causes vomiting and diarrhea 1 to 8 hours after a food allergen is ingested. It often develops during the first year of life when solids are introduced, and the foods most commonly associated with FPIES are milk, soy, and grains.

Food Allergy Testing

If you notice a reaction to any food in your baby, never try to diagnose it yourself. Among other risks, this can lead to the unnecessary elimination of healthy foods. A board-certified allergist will consider several factors and rule out other unrelated health conditions before making a diagnosis. Of enormous help to your pediatrician and allergist is your careful tracking and recording of any physical reactions that you think may be related to certain foods. This is particularly important when you are dealing with less common food allergies that do not involve IgE antibodies. I've included a food-reaction tracking tool on pages 116 and 117 to help make this process easier.

If your child is at risk for developing food allergies, your doctor may recommend introducing the top allergens after some additional testing in the office first (and potentially before your child is 6 months old). Here are several standardized medical tests that can help diagnose food allergies:

- **Skin Prick Test:** An initial screening for food allergies is often performed using a skin prick test, which measures the presence of IgE antibodies for a certain food. Using a very small needle, diluted amounts of the food in question are "pricked" into the skin, which is then monitored for 15 to 30 minutes. A "wheal" or red bump that develops on the skin at the site of the prick may indicate an allergy to the food, at which point further testing is advised, as skin prick tests do carry a high rate of false positives.
- **Blood Test:** Blood tests can measure the immune system's response to certain foods by checking for IgE antibodies. The higher the level of antibodies, the higher the likelihood of an allergy to the food. If both the skin prick test and the blood test are positive, a food allergy is usually assumed.
- **Oral Food Challenge:** Considered the gold standard in food allergy diagnosis, oral food challenges must be performed under the supervision of a doctor. The patient is given small, increasing amounts of the food in question and monitored carefully for symptoms. If no symptoms are observed, the challenge is repeated but with a larger dose.

Peanut Allergies

Peanut is the most common food allergen. The recommendations for introducing peanut are broken down into three groups, roughly based on risk according to the LEAP study, published in the *New England Journal of Medicine* in 2015:

1. If your baby has severe eczema, an egg allergy, or both, consult with your pediatrician or allergist, who will likely first recommend an allergy blood test or a skin prick test. Depending on the results, your doctor will advise you on whether and how to introduce peanut foods between the ages of 4 to 6 months, either at home or under the supervision of a health-care professional.

2. If your baby has mild to moderate eczema, peanut foods may be introduced at around 6 months of age at home or under the supervision of a health-care professional in order to reduce the risk of developing a peanut allergy.

3. If your baby does not have eczema or food allergies, you can introduce peanut foods at home in an age-appropriate way, along with other solids, from the age of 6 months.

If your pediatrician has advised that you introduce peanut foods at home, there are a few ways to safely do so. Once your baby has successfully tried a few new foods, find a time when your baby is healthy and you know you will be home and fully attentive for at least 2 hours, so that you can watch for any potential reactions. (Your pediatrician will be grateful if you do this on a weekday and in the morning.) The key is to offer about 2 grams of peanut protein, which is equivalent to 2 teaspoons of peanut butter. However, peanut butter and whole peanuts are choking hazards. The three following preparations are infant-safe options for offering peanut the BLW way:

1. Thinly spread 2 teaspoons of peanut butter on strips of toast.

2. Stir 2 teaspoons of peanut butter into oatmeal and offer on a preloaded spoon.

3. Measure 2 teaspoons of smooth peanut butter or peanut flour into a small bowl, add 2 to 3 teaspoons of hot water or warmed breast milk, and stir until the mixture is well blended and thinned. Once it has cooled, mix it with a little infant cereal or another food your baby enjoys and offer it on a preloaded spoon.

Only offer peanut foods (and other common allergens) alongside foods your baby has eaten before so that you can clearly identify the cause of any potential reaction. Offer only one bite of the peanut food at first. After the first bite, wait 10 minutes. If there is no allergic reaction, offer the rest and then continue to offer peanut foods in an infant-safe way at least three times a week going forward.

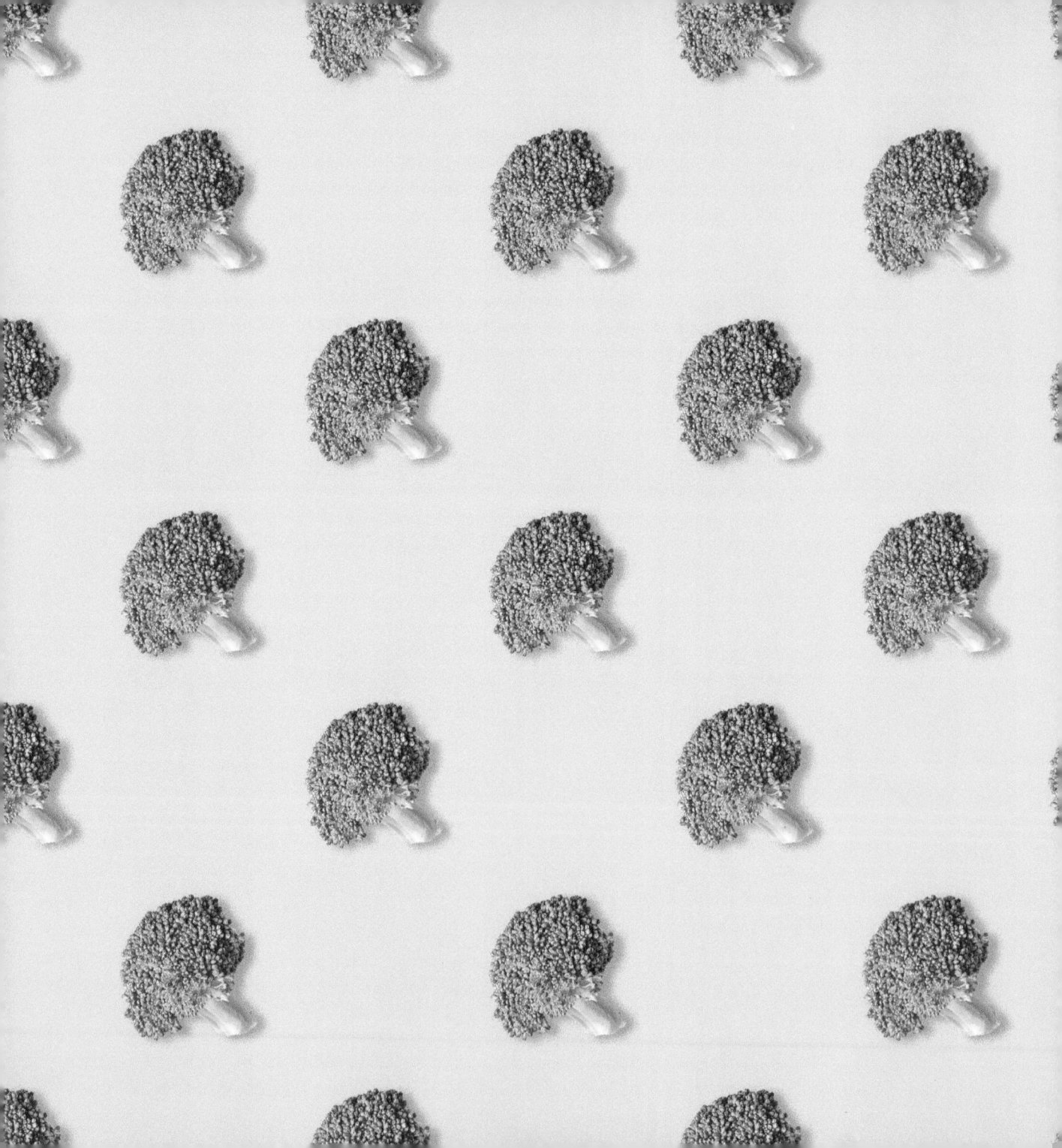

CHAPTER SEVEN

FOOD INTOLERANCES & SENSITIVITIES

ood intolerances are often confused with food allergies because the symptoms can look and feel similar. Whereas food allergies are caused by the immune system, food intolerances are usually triggered by an inability to process or digest certain foods. Common symptoms include cramping, gas, bloating, nausea, diarrhea, and constipation.

Although they are uncomfortable, food intolerances and sensitivities are not life-threatening and can happen in response to many triggers, such as food additives, preservatives, artificial colors, and a type of natural fiber called inulin, which is found in foods like onions and Brussels sprouts. Lactose intolerance happens when the body lacks the enzymes needed to break down lactose, a natural sugar found in milk. Celiac disease is not considered a food allergy, as it is an autoimmune disease whereby gluten causes the immune system to react in a way that leads to intestinal inflammation and malabsorption.

Some people with pollen allergies can have mild reactions to certain raw fruits and vegetables. This is called oral allergy syndrome. Although it is not a true food allergy, it can cause itching and swelling in the mouth and is usually a lifelong condition, although it is not life-threatening. The best way to avoid oral allergy syndrome is to avoid handling those particular foods. The peels of such fruits and vegetables generally cause a greater reaction than the flesh, and some people experience less of a reaction when the food is peeled, cooked, or canned.

Symptoms of Food Sensitivity in Babies

Sometimes a baby may be sensitive to certain foods. Symptoms such as rash, wheezing, diarrhea, and vomiting may indicate a problem with food, but they are also common signs of viral infection or other nonfood-related conditions.

As their immune and digestive systems mature over time, most babies will not have food-related issues. To be on the safe side, take note of any reactions you believe are related to foods. If you notice that a specific food is causing a significant or ongoing reaction, contact your pediatrician to discuss your concerns. In the back of this book, you will find a list of tummy-friendly food swaps you can make to help manage this process, as well as a food-reaction tracking tool to help you keep notes on your baby's progress.

You may have noticed after starting your baby on solids that the color, consistency, and odor of your baby's stool has changed, and your baby may have more gas than usual. This is normal and does not necessarily indicate a food sensitivity. Over time, your baby's digestive system will adjust to solid foods and these symptoms will reduce or disappear.

Baby Gas

Gas is a very normal part of babyhood and has a variety of causes, which include swallowing air (while eating, drinking, or sucking a pacifier), excessive crying, starting solids, new foods, a still-developing digestive tract, viruses, and minor digestive issues such as constipation.

Gas does not seem to bother most babies. Others may be uncomfortable, restless, upset, or even incensed until it passes, but gas is not generally dangerous.

Most of the time, baby gas does not mean anything is wrong. In fact, gas is not considered a medical condition but rather a temporary, usually minor symptom. Nonetheless, the disproportionately huge sounds coming from a small baby can certainly seem alarming at times! If your baby has started solids and you are concerned about an increase in gas and worried that it is making your baby uncomfortable, here is what you need to know:

1. If your baby has minor amounts of gas (and is generally happy but gets a little fussy before passing gas), there is no need to see your pediatrician. Just make a note and bring it up at your baby's next appointment.

2. Gentle belly massage, pumping your baby's legs in a bicycle pedaling motion, doing tummy time, and warm baths can all help alleviate discomfort.

3. Over time and as your baby's digestive system matures, gas usually becomes less of a problem.

4. Although babies (and adults for that matter) vary in their responses to different foods, some foods may cause more gas than others, such as beans, legumes, cabbage, broccoli, cauliflower, stone and citrus fruits, bran, and oatmeal. If you feel certain foods are causing excess gas, it might be tempting to cut them out of your baby's diet. Know that eliminating them does not always help, and these types of nutrient-dense, fiber-rich foods are important components of a healthy diet that you do not want your baby to miss.

5. If you are still concerned, use the food-reaction tracking tool in the back of this book to record foods that you think may be causing extra gas and discuss them with your doctor. For some babies, excessive gas can be a sign of a food sensitivity.

6. In rare cases, gas can signal a more serious digestive issue. If your baby experiences increased gas along with excessive fussiness, vomiting, constipation, bloody stools, or a fever of 100.4 degrees Fahrenheit (38 degrees Celsius) or higher, call your pediatrician right away.

You Are Ready to Try Baby-Led Weaning!

In the end, much of baby-led feeding (and parenting in general, for that matter) comes down to trust—in both yourself as the expert on your baby and in your baby's own ability to self-feed, self-regulate, and self-nourish. My hope is that you will use the guidance and information in this book to partner with your baby throughout the adventures of BLW and carry these practices with you throughout your child's life. For your little one, this tender introduction to food is only the beginning! Think of your baby's wonder at the first taste of mango or strawberry—that face full of smiles.

Some of the greatest lifelong gifts you can give your child are an affinity for healthy foods, a taste for flavor, an appreciation of texture, and a capacity to experience the profound connectedness between food and love. Enjoy food as a family activity and as a pleasure that brings you closer, helps you communicate, celebrates your culture, and nourishes you in multiple, lasting ways. Good luck and relish each moment of the fantastic journey ahead!

FOOD REACTION TRACKER

FOOD	DATE/TIME	DESCRIPTION OF REACTION/ SYMPTOMS	HOW LONG AFTER EATING THE FOOD DID THE REACTION OR SYMPTOMS APPEAR?

HOW MUCH OF THE FOOD WAS EATEN TO CAUSE THE REACTION?	DOES THE REACTION OR SYMPTOM OCCUR EVERY TIME THE FOOD IS EATEN?	DURATION OF REACTION	HOW DID YOU RESPOND, AND DID IT HELP?

ALLERGY SWAPS

If you discover that your baby has a food allergy, this list of alternatives can help ensure that eliminating the allergen does not mean leaving important nutrients out of your baby's diet. Foods in the right-hand column offer many of the same nutrients as the foods in the left-hand column. For example, if your baby is allergic to soy, offer lentils instead, both of which offer many of the same nutrients.

ALLERGY	SWAP
Peanut butter or other, tree-nut butters	Sunflower seed butter or tahini (sesame paste)
Egg	The following options can be used as a substitute for 1 egg when cooking and baking: Mix 1 tablespoon of chia seeds with 3 tablespoons of water, and let it sit for 5 minutes or until the mixture forms a gel; or 1 teaspoon of yeast dissolved in 1/4 cup of warm water; or 1 tablespoon of ground flaxseed mixed with 2 tablespoons of warm water, allowed to sit for 5 minutes until it forms a gel; or 2 tablespoons of blended tofu; or mix 1 ½ tablespoons of water with 1 ½ tablespoons oil (such as avocado oil) and 1 teaspoon baking powder
Meat	Beans, legumes, tofu, nut butters, poultry, fish, shellfish
Cow's milk	Soy or pea milk
Cow's milk yogurt	Coconut yogurt, soy yogurt
Fish	Meat, poultry, flaxseeds, walnuts, shellfish, chia seeds, hemp hearts
Shellfish	Fish, meat, poultry, flaxseed, walnuts, chia seeds, hemp hearts
Soy	Beans, lentils
Wheat	Oats, quinoa, brown rice, millet, buckwheat, amaranth, teff, corn

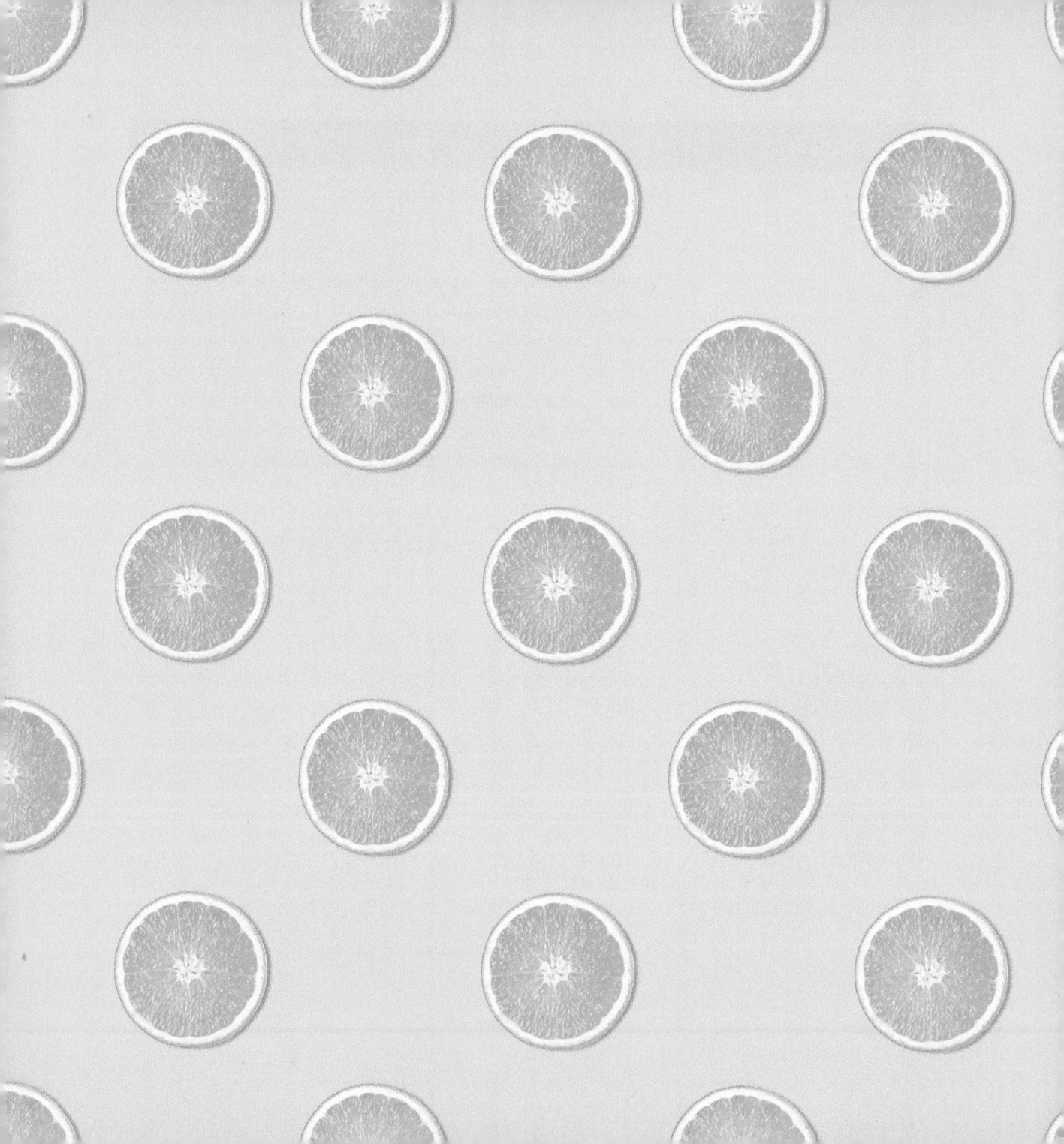

REFERENCES

Ajenifuja, Bolaji. "Weaning Practices in Developing Countries." In *Weaning: Why, What, and When?*, edited by Angel Ballabriga and Jean Rey, 205–10. New York: Raven Press, 1987.

Alvisi, Patrizia, Sandra Brusa, Stefano Alboresi, Sergio Amarri, Paolo Bottau, Giovanni Cavagni, Barbara Corrandini, et al. "Recommendations on Complementary Feeding for Healthy, Full-Term Infants." *Italian Journal of Pediatrics* 41, no. 36 (April 2015). doi.org/10.1186/s13052-015-0143-5.

American Academy of Pediatrics. "Infant Food and Feeding." Accessed October 21, 2019. https://www.aap.org/en-us/advocacy-and-policy/aap-health-initiatives /HALF-Implementation-Guide/Age-Specific-Content/Pages/Infant-Food-and -Feeding.aspx.

American Academy of Pediatrics Committee on Nutrition. "Food Allergy." *In Pediatric Nutrition*, 7th ed., edited by Ronald E. Kleinman and Frank R. Greer, 845–62. Elk Grove Village, IL: American Academy of Pediatrics, 2014.

The American National Red Cross. *Pediatric First Aid/CPR/AED: Ready Reference.* 2011. https://www.redcross.org/content/dam/redcross/atg/PDF_s/Health___Safety _Services/Training/Pediatric_ready_reference.pdf.

Anabrees, Jasim, Flavia Indrio, Bosco Paes, and Khalid Al Faleh. "Probiotics for Infantile Colic: A Systematic Review." *BMC Pediatrics* 13, no. 186 (November 2013). doi.org /10.1186/1471-2431-13-186.

Applegate, Catherine C., Joe Rowles, Katherine Ranard, Sookyoung Jeon, and John W. Erdman. "Soy Consumption and the Risk of Prostate Cancer: An Updated Systematic Review and Meta-Analysis." *Nutrients* 10, no. 1 (January 2018): 40. doi.org/10.3390 /nu10010040.

Berchelmann, Kathleen. "The Benefits and Tricks to Having a Family Dinner." *Healthy-children.org*. Last modified December 30, 2015. https://www.healthychildren.org/English/family-life/family-dynamics/Pages/Mealtime-as-Family-Time.aspx.

Bourn, Diane, and John Prescott. "A Comparison of the Nutritional Value, Sensory Qualities, and Food Safety of Organically and Conventionally Produced Foods." *Critical Reviews in Food Science and Nutrition* 42, no. 1 (January 2002): 1–34. doi.org/10.1080/10408690290825439.

Brooks, Megan. "FDA Clears First Epinephrine Autoinjector for Infants." *Medscape*. November 21, 2017. https://www.medscape.com/viewarticle/889007.

Brown, Amy E. "No Difference in Self-Reported Frequency of Choking Between Infants Introduced to Solid Foods Using a Baby-Led Weaning or Traditional Spoon-Feeding Approach." *Journal of Human Nutrition and Dietetics* 31, no. 4 (December 2017): 496–504. doi.org/10.1111/jhn.12528.

Centers for Disease Control and Prevention. "Burden of Foodborne Illness: Findings." The website of the Centers for Disease Control and Prevention. Last modified November 5, 2018. https://www.cdc.gov/foodborneburden/2011-foodborne-estimates.html.

Chi, Feng, Rong Wu, Yue-Can Zeng, Rui Xing, Yang Liu, and Zhao-Guo Xu. "Post-Diagnosis Soy Food Intake and Breast Cancer Survival: A Meta-Analysis of Cohort Studies." *Asian Pacific Journal of Cancer Prevention* 14, no. 4 (April 2013): 2407–12. doi.org/10.7314/APJCP.2013.14.4.2407.

Committee to Review the Dietary Reference Intakes for Sodium and Potassium. "Sodium: Dietary Reference Intakes for Adequacy." In *Dietary Reference Intakes for Sodium and Potassium*, edited by Virginia A. Stallings, Meghan Harrison, and Maria Oria. Washington, DC: The National Academies Press, 2019. https://www.nap.edu/read/25353/chapter/13#236.

Daniels, L., Heath, A.M., Williams, S.M. *et al*. Baby-Led Introduction to SolidS (BLISS) study: a randomised controlled trial of a baby-led approach to complementary feeding. *BMC Pediatr* 15, 179 (2015) doi:10.1186/s12887-015-0491-8.

Du Toit, George, Graham Roberts, Peter H. Sayre, Henry T. Bahnson, Suzana Radulovic, Alexandra F. Santos, Helen A. Brough, et al. "Randomized Trial of Peanut Consumption in Infants at Risk for Peanut Allergy." *New England Journal of Medicine* 372, no. 9 (February 2015): 803–13. doi.org/10.1056/NEJMoa1414850.

Erickson, Liz Williams, Rachael Taylor, Jillian Haszard, Elizabeth A. Fleming, Lisa Daniels, Brittany J. Morison, Claudia Leong, et al. "Impact of a Modified Version of Baby-Led Weaning on Infant Food and Nutrient Intakes: The BLISS Randomized Controlled Trial." *Nutrients* 10, no. 6 (June 2018): 740. doi.org/10.3390/nu10060740.

Fangupo, Louise J., Anne-Louise M. Heath, Sheila M. Williams, Liz W. Erickson Williams, Brittany J. Morison, Elizabeth Ann Fleming, Barry J. Taylor, et al. "A Baby-Led Approach to Eating Solids and Risk of Choking." *Pediatrics* 138, no. 4 (October 2016). doi.org/10.1542/peds.2016-0772.

Food Allergy Research and Education (FARE). "Facts and Statistics." The website of Food Allergy Research and Education (FARE). Accessed October 21, 2019. https://www.foodallergy.org/life-with-food-allergies/food-allergy-101/facts-and-statistics.

Food Allergy Research and Education (FARE). "Symptoms of an Allergic Reaction to Food." The website of Food Allergy Research and Education (FARE). Accessed October 21, 2019. https://www.foodallergy.org/life-with-food-allergies/food-allergy-101/symptoms-of-an-allergic-reaction-to-food.

Greer, Frank R., Scott H. Sicherer, and A. Wesley Burks. "The Effects of Early Nutritional Interventions on the Development of Atopic Disease in Infants and Children: The Role of Maternal Dietary Restriction, Breastfeeding, Hydrolyzed Formulas, and Timing of Introduction of Allergenic Complementary Foods." *Pediatrics* 143, no. 4 (April 2019): e20190281. doi.org/10.1542/peds.2019-0281.

Gupta, Ruchi S., Christopher M. Warren, Bridget M. Smith, Jesse A. Blumenstock, Jialing Jiang, Matthew M. Davis, and Kari C. Nadeau. "The Public Health Impact of Parent-Reported Childhood Food Allergies in the United States." *Pediatrics* 142, no. 6 (December 2018): e20181235. doi.org/10.1542/peds.2018-1235.

Hamilton-Reeves, Jill M., Gabriela Vazquez-Benitez, Sue J. Duval, William R. Phipps, Mindy S. Kurzer, and Mark J. Messina. "Clinical Studies Show No Effects of Soy Protein or Isoflavones on Reproductive Hormones in Men: Results of a Meta-Analysis." *Fertility and Sterility* 94, no. 3 (August 2010): 997–1007. doi.org/10.1016/j.fertnstert .2009.04.038.

Hammons, Amber J., and Barbara H. Fiese. "Is Frequency of Shared Family Meals Related to the Nutritional Health of Children and Adolescents?" *Pediatrics* 127, no. 6 (June 2011): e1565–74. doi.org/10.1542/peds.2010-1440.

Helwig, Jenna. *Baby-Led Feeding*. Boston: Houghton Mifflin, 2019.

Howcroft, Rachel. "Weaned Upon a Time. Studies of the Infant Diet in Prehistory." PhD diss., Stockholm University, 2013. https://pdfs.semanticscholar.org/da28 /dc0fb248cd8ed8580431afa7180a89b6d2e5.pdf.

Jackson, Kristen D., LaJeana D. Howie, and Lara J. Akinbami. *Trends in Allergic Conditions Among Children: United States, 1997–2011*. NCHS Data Brief, no. 121, 2013. https://www.cdc.gov/nchs/data/databriefs/db121.pdf.

Lee, Gwenyth O'Neill, Maribel Paredes Olortegui, Sylvia Rengifo Pinedo, Ramya Ambikapathi, Pablo Penataro Yori, Margaret Kosek, and Laura E. Caulfield. "Infant Feeding Practices in the Peruvian Amazon: Implications for Programs to Improve Feeding." *Pan American Journal of Public Health* 36, no. 3 (September 2014): 150–7. https://www.ncbi.nlm.nih.gov/pubmed/25418764.

Lessen, Rachelle, and Katherine F. Kavanagh. "Position of the Academy of Nutrition and Dietetics: Promoting and Supporting Breastfeeding." *Journal of the Academy of Nutrition and Dietetics* 115, no. 3 (March 2015): 444–9. doi.org/10.1016/j.jand .2014.12.014.

Melina, Vesanto, Winston Craig, and Susan Levin. "Position of the Academy of Nutrition and Dietetics: Vegetarian Diets." *Journal of the Academy of Nutrition and Dietetics* 116, no. 12 (December 2016): 1970–80. doi.org/10.1016/j.jand.2016.09.025.

Messina, Mark, and Geoffrey Redmond. "Effects of Soy Protein and Soybean Isoflavones on Thyroid Function in Healthy Adults and Hypothyroid Patients: A Review of the Relevant Literature." *Thyroid* 16, no. 3 (April 2006): 249–58. doi.org/10.1089/thy.2006.16.249.

Mie, Axel, Helle Raun Andersen, Stefan Gunnarsson, Johannes Kahl, Emmanuelle Kesse-Guyot, Ewa Rembiałkowska, Gianluca Quaglio, and Philippe Grandjean. "Human Health Implications of Organic Food and Organic Agriculture: A Comprehensive Review." *Environmental Health* 16, no. 1 (October 2017): 111. doi.org/10.1186/s12940-017-0315-4.

Morison, Brittany, Rachael Taylor, Jillian J. Haszard, Claire J. Schramm, Liz Williams Erickson, Louise J. Fangupo, Elizabeth A. Fleming, et al. "How Different Are Baby-Led Weaning and Conventional Complementary Feeding? A Cross-Sectional Study of Infants Aged 6–8 Months." *BMJ Open* 6, no. 5 (May 2016): e010665. doi.org/10.1136/bmjopen-2015-010665.

Murdoch Children's Research Institute. "Probiotics for Infants and Children." Fact sheet. Melbourne: Centre for Community Child Health, the Royal Children's Hospital Melbourne, 2014. https://www.rch.org.au/uploadedfiles/main/content/ccch/cpr_vol22_no1_factsheet.pdf.

The National Academies of Sciences, Engineering, Medicine. *Dietary Reference Intakes for Sodium and Potassium: Consensus Study Report.* PowerPoint presentation, 2019. http://www.nationalacademies.org/hmd/~/media/Files/Report%20Files/2019/Dietary-Reference-Intakes/webinar-slides.pdf.

National Institute of Allergy and Infectious Diseases. *Guidelines for the Diagnosis and Management of Food Allergy in the United States: Summary for Patients, Families, and Caregivers.* Washington, DC: National Institutes of Health, 2011. https://www.niaid.nih.gov/sites/default/files/faguidelinespatient.pdf.

National Institutes of Health. "Choking—Infant Under 1 Year." The website of MedlinePlus and the ADAM Medical Encyclopedia. Updated September 11, 2019. https://medlineplus.gov/ency/article/000048.htm.

Pan American Health Organization and World Health Organization. *Guiding Principles for Complementary Feeding of the Breastfed Child*. Washington, DC: World Health Organization, 2003. https://www.who.int/nutrition/publications/guiding_principles _compfeeding_breastfed.pdf.

Rapley, Gill, and Tracey Murkett. *Baby-Led Weaning: Helping Your Baby to Love Good Food*. London: Vermilion, 2008.

Satter, Ellyn. "Division of Responsibility in Feeding." The website of the Ellyn Satter Institute. Accessed October 21, 2019. https://www.ellynsatterinstitute.org/how-to -feed/the-division-of-responsibility-in-feeding/.

Schilling, Leslie, and Wendy Jo Peterson. *Born to Eat: Whole, Healthy Foods from Baby's First Bite*. New York: Skyhorse, 2017.

Smith-Spangler, Crystal, Margaret L. Brandeau, Grace E. Hunter, J. Clay Bavinger, Maren Pearson, Paul J. Eschbach, Vandana Sundaram, et al. "Are Organic Foods Safer or Healthier Than Conventional Alternatives?: A Systematic Review." *Annals of Internal Medicine* 157, no. 5 (September 2012): 348–66. doi.org/10.7326/0003-4819-157-5 -201209040-00007.

Tate, Julie F. "Feeding Practices of Mothers in the Gobi Desert of Mongolia." MS thesis, East Tennessee State University, 2011. https://dc.etsu.edu/etd/1228.

Taylor, Rachael W., Sheila Williams, Louise J. Fangupo, Benjamin John Wheeler, Barry J. Taylor, Lisa Daniels, Elizabeth A. Fleming, et al. "Effect of a Baby-Led Approach to Complementary Feeding on Infant Growth and Overweight: A Randomized Clinical Trial." *JAMA Pediatrics* 171, no. 9 (September 2017): 838–46. doi.org/10.1001/jama pediatrics.2017.1284.

Togias, Alkis, Susan F. Cooper, Maria L. Acebal, Amal Assa'ad, James R. Baker, Lisa A. Beck, Julie Block, et al. *Addendum Guidelines for the Prevention of Peanut Allergy in the United States: Report of the National Institute of Allergy and Infectious Diseases-Sponsored Expert Panel*. Bethesda, MD: National Institute of Allergy and Infectious Diseases, 2016. https://www.niaid.nih.gov/sites/default/files /addendum-peanut-allergy-prevention-guidelines.pdf.

Townsend Ellen, Nicola Pitchford. "Baby Knows Best? The Impact of Weaning Style on Food Preferences and Body Mass Index in Early Childhood in a Case–Controlled Sample." *BMJ Open* 2, no. 1 (January 2012): e000298. doi.org/10.1136/bmjopen-2011-000298.

Trasande, Leonardo, Rachel M. Shaffer, Sheela Sathyanarayana, and Council on Environmental Health. "Food Additives and Child Health." *Pediatrics* 142, no. 2 (August 2018): e20181408. doi.org/10.1542/peds.2018-1408.

United States Department of Agriculture. "'Danger Zone' (40°F–140°F)." Food safety fact sheet. Updated June 28, 2017. https://www.fsis.usda.gov/wps/portal/fsis/topics/food-safety-education/get-answers/food-safety-fact-sheets/safe-food-handling/danger-zone-40-f-140-f/CT_Index.

United States Department of Agriculture. "Safe Minimum Internal Temperature Chart." Food safety fact sheet. Updated May 6, 2019. https://www.fsis.usda.gov/wps/portal/fsis/topics/food-safety-education/get-answers/food-safety-fact-sheets/safe-food-handling/safe-minimum-internal-temperature-chart/ct_index.

Van der Horst, Klazine, and Ester F. C. Sleddens. "Parenting Styles, Feeding Styles and Food-Related Parenting Practices in Relation to Toddlers' Eating Styles: A Cluster-Analytic Approach." *PLOS ONE* 12, no. 5 (May 2017): e0178149. doi.org/10.1371/journal.pone.0178149.

Woo Baidal, Jennifer A., Lindsey Locks, Erika R. Cheng, Tiffany L. Blake-Lamb, Meghan E. Perkins, and Elsie M. Taveras. "Risk Factors for Childhood Obesity in the First 1,000 Days: A Systematic Review." *American Journal of Preventive Medicine* 50, no. 6 (February 2016): 761–79. doi.org/10.1016/j.amepre.2015.11.012.

World Health Organization. "Complementary Feeding." Accessed August 26, 2019. https://www.who.int/nutrition/topics/complementary_feeding/en/.

Zhao, Xin Yuan, Edgar Chambers, Ziad Matta, Thomas M. Loughin, and Edward E. Carey. "Consumer Sensory Analysis of Organically and Conventionally Grown Vegetables." *Journal of Food Science* 72, no. 2 (March 2007): S87–S91. doi.org/10.1111/j.1750-3841.2007.00277.x.

INDEX

Parmesan, 39, 61
    soft, cream and, 67, 75, 85, 94
chicken/turkey, 51
choking hazards, 28–29, 75, 91, 95, 108
citrus, 71, 114

D

delayed food allergies, 106

E

eczema, 104–105, 108
eggs
    BLW menu options, 22
    egg allergies, 102, 103, 108
    egg substitutes, 119
    food thermometer, testing egg preparations with, 36
    in French toast, 77
    iron content of, 38, 57
    nutrients in, 58
    omega-3 enriched eggs, as recommended, 57
    raw eggs, handling safely, 35

F

fish, 4, 22, 35, 55, 58, 103, 119
Food Allergy Research and Education (FARE), 103
food groups, three, 38
food intolerance, symptoms of, 112
Food Protein-Induced Enterocolitis Syndrome (FPIES), 106
food sensitivity, symptoms of, 113
food swaps, maintaining nutrients, 118–119
foodborne illness, dangers of, 32–34

foods to avoid, list of, 95
formula feeding
    baby cereals, not replacing, 88
    during baby's cold or illness, 19
    cow's milk, not supplanting, 94
    in the first year, 38, 41
    meals, timing after feedings, 18
    shifting recommendations on, 4
    transitioning from, 1, 14–15
French toast, 28, 38, 77
fruits, 38, 61, 67, 69, 71, 72, 78, 95

G

gag reflex, gagging and, 29, 30–31
gas, gastrointestinal conditions and, 34, 82, 106, 113–114
grains, whole, 4, 15, 49, 77, 87
green beans, 39, 65

H

Helwig, Jenna, 11
honey, infant botulism and, 94, 96
Howcroft, Rachel, 4
hummus, 39, 45, 49, 75
hungry cues, learn to recognize, 5, 7, 14

I

iron, important nutrient for overall health, 8, 38, 41, 45, 94

K

kiwi, 39, 69

L

Learning Early About Peanut Allergy (LEAP), 104, 108

M

mandarin orange, 38, 71
mango, 11, 38, 49, 115
meat, 22, 28–29, 33, 51, 53, 91, 94, 119
milk
    coconut milk, 49
    cow's milk, 94, 118, 119
    FPIES, associated with, 106
    in French toast, 77
    lactose intolerance, 112
    milk feedings in BLW meal schedule, 15
    oatmeal, cooking in milk, 87
    as a top allergen, 102, 103
Murkett, Tracey, 4

N

National Institute of Allergy and Infectious Diseases, 102, 104
nutrients for development
    choline, 45, 57, 58
    iron, 8, 38, 41, 45, 49, 61
    zinc, 49, 58, 87
nutrients to limit, 75, 78, 96
nuts, nut butters and, 15, 49, 67, 75, 91, 95, 108, 119

O

oatmeal, 49, 87, 91, 108, 114
oral allergy syndrome, 112
oral food challenge, allergies and, 107
organic food. See produce, organic or conventional

ACKNOWLEDGMENTS

Many thanks to my wonderful editors Morgan Shanahan, Anne Lowrey, and Erika Sloan, as well as the entire team at Callisto.

I am forever grateful to Sherry Coleman Collins, MS, RDN, LD; Dr. Jennifer Gruen, MD; Dr. Michael D. Wolf, PhD; Peter Acker, MD; Liz Weiss, MS, RDN; Dr. Steven Koutroupas, MD; and Cindy Linkas for their expertise and boundless generosity in reviewing this manuscript.

Thank you to my village—Jennifer and Jeff Enslin, Jackie and Chris Schiavone, Jodi and Daniel Kaderabek, Bettina and Nik Nackley, Jennifer O'Hara, Mary McCarthy, Erin and Jeff Cast, Liz and Brian Woods, Natalie Blundell, Toby Amidor, Francesca Mercurio, Amy Brennan, Vicki Downs, Serena Jones, Meghan DiPerna, and all my other dear friends who have supported me through the thick, the thin, and everything in between.

The hugest forever thanks to Leslie Casillas for her daily love, support, and healthy, delicious food.

To my brother and his wife, Chris and Danielle Linkas, for always helping me find my true north.

Deepest thanks to my most wonderful parents, Tom and Cindy Linkas, who imprinted me early on with a lifelong appreciation for the connection between food and love.

And to my girls . . . my three sweet girls, who made me a mother. Thank you for providing most of the inspiration for this book, and all of the inspiration for my life. I love you.

ABOUT THE AUTHOR

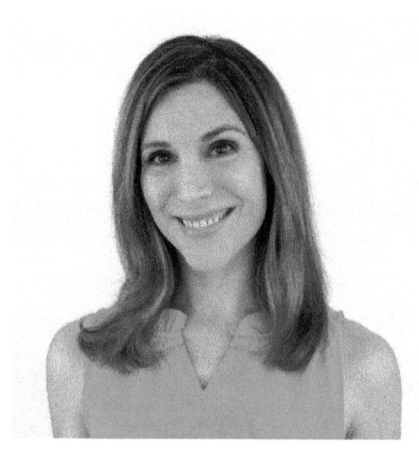

Malina Linkas Malkani, MS, RDN, CDN, is a registered dietitian nutritionist and trusted nutrition expert in local and national media outlets and publications including *U.S. News & World Report, Sirius XM Doctor Radio, Forbes, Newsweek, Reader's Digest, Insider, HuffPost,* CNN, and Food Network.

Malina owns a nutrition lifestyle company and private practice (www.MalinaMalkani.com), dedicated to providing parents with tools, kid-friendly recipes, and programs that make it easier to feed the entire family a mostly plant-based, nutrient-dense, whole-food diet (that they will actually eat). Her mission is to reshape the nutritional habits and behaviors of our next generation to optimize their long-term health and reduce the likelihood of obesity, cancer, and chronic lifestyle diseases.

She is also the Director of Nutrition at Rejuvenan Global Health, a personalized digital health platform based in Manhattan, New York, offering clinical wellness, on-demand telemedicine, and virtual primary care. A former educator with KIDS' FANS (Fitness and Nutrition Services) at Stamford Hospital in Connecticut, Malina has served as a national media spokesperson for the Academy of Nutrition and Dietetics, earned the Commission on Dietetic Registration's two certificates of training in adult weight management (Levels 1 and 2), and completed her dietetic internship at the accredited James J. Peters VA Medical Center in the Bronx, New York, where she subsequently worked as an outpatient weight loss and bariatric surgery dietitian.

She completed her undergraduate degrees at Northwestern University and earned a master's degree in clinical nutrition from New York University. A single mom of three young girls, Malina currently resides outside of New York City. When she's not working, she can usually be found running around with her kids, cooking, hanging out on Instagram (@healthy.mom.healthy.kids), or making music.

CPSIA information can be obtained
at www.ICGtesting.com
Printed in the USA
LVHW020832291120
672911LV00007B/13